Contents

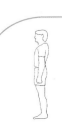

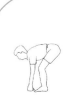

11 User feedback on these guidelines

Appendices

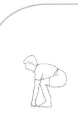

Acknowledgements

The Guideline Development Group (GDG) would like to acknowledge the following people who have contributed to the development of these guidelines.

Professor Julius Sim, Professor of Health Care Research, Keele University, for advice on defining consensus and the level of consensus necessary to make a recommendation.

Dr Nadine Foster, Senior Lecturer in Therapies (pain management), Primary Care Musculoskeletal Research Centre, Keele University, for section 8 on implementation.

Andrea Peace, Library and Information Services Manager, Chartered Society of Physiotherapy (CSP), for ongoing support during the development of these guidelines.

Samantha Molloy, Information Services Librarian, CSP, for the literature searches in both 2003 and 2005 and the literature search strategy (appendix C).

Linda Griffiths, Information Services Librarian, CSP, for ongoing support during the development of these guidelines.

Alison Jinks, Library Assistant, CSP, for organising the ordering of articles for the literature review and data verification.

Sharlene Ting, Project Worker, CSP, for her work on the systematic reviews.

Jenni Davies, Project worker, CSP, for her work on the systematic reviews.

Anna Luce, Research Associate, Nursing, Midwifery and Allied Health Professions Research Unit, Northumbria University, for her contribution to the systematic review.

Dawn Wheeler, Head of Research and Clinical Effectiveness, for her support to the CSP guidelines team and her work on this project.

The Clinical Guidelines Endorsement Panel (CGEP) and the reviewers for their constructive comments. Actions following this improved the quality of this final document.

Ceri Sedgley, Project Officer, CSP, for editing this document and developing the audit pack.

Publications unit for design and production.

All other CSP staff who advised and supported the team.

Outline of the clinical guidelines for the physiotherapy management of persistent LBP

Clinical guidelines considering all aspects of the physiotherapy management of people with persistent LBP would be an extremely large and impractical document. This topic has been sub divided into 2 guidelines. Part 1 Exercise and Part 2 Manual Therapy. This was a pragmatic decision made for the following reasons:

- publication of each part, would be quicker and provide access to up to date knowledge
- each part of these guidelines would be a convenient size for users
- future updating of these guidelines can be done for each part separately thus making this process manageable.

Two systematic reviews, associated with these guidelines are being prepared for publication in peer reviewed journals. Their working titles at the time of writing are:

- A systematic review and synthesis of higher quality evidence of the effectiveness of exercise interventions for non-specific low back pain of at least six weeks duration
- A hands-on approach for sub-acute and chronic low back pain; a systematic review and synthesis of best evidence on the effectiveness of massage, mobilisation and manipulation

A quick reference guide is attached to the back cover of each document and can be torn off for easy reference.

The accompanying audit pack is inserted in the front cover pocket of the exercise section.

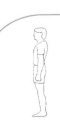

Executive summary

These guidelines apply to people between 18 and 65 years of age with persistent low back pain (LBP), which is of musculoskeletal origin, emanates from the lumbar spine, and has lasted for six weeks or more. The recommendations for practice are intended to assist physiotherapists and people with LBP in making decisions about whether to exercise and which type of exercise to pursue after physiotherapy assessment.

Persistent LBP was identified by Chartered Society of Physiotherapy (CSP) members as a priority area for clinical guidelines in 2002[1] and a guideline development group (GDG) was formed of expert clinicians, researchers and a representative of the patient perspective. The GDG's focus was to investigate whether a range of exercises frequently used by physiotherapists (i.e., mobilising, strengthening, aerobic, general, core stability, hydrotherapy, McKenzie*) were effective in reducing pain, and improving both function and psychological status. A systematic review of the literature was the basis for the recommendations thus ensuring their foundation on relevant and high quality research evidence. Where there were gaps in the literature, a nominal group consensus technique was used to generate consensus evidence from a wider expert group that included the GDG. By expert consensus, the GDG made a range of recommendations. These guidelines were peer reviewed prior to their endorsement and publication.

Recommendations for practice

The key clinical recommendation is that:

> People with persistent LBP should be given the opportunity to participate in an exercise programme, in a form appropriate and acceptable to each individual, after physiotherapy assessment.

The GDG recommend mobilising, strengthening, organised aerobic, general, core stability, hydrotherapy and McKenzie exercises to improve function. And mobilising, strengthening, organised aerobic, general, hydrotherapy and McKenzie exercises to reduce pain and improve psychological status.

Recommendations for research

The key research question is:

> Are there identifiable sub-groups of people with persistent LBP who respond best to particular types of exercise?

Conclusion

These guidelines are a valuable tool for physiotherapists in clinical practice, for people with persistent LBP, and those involved in planning, funding and carrying out research studies. The recommendations are based on the best available evidence but as new evidence emerges these recommendations should be reviewed. A formal update to these guidelines is planned for 2011.

* see section 4.2 for definition of McKenzie exercises

1 Introduction and background

1.1 Definition of persistent low back pain

Persistent LBP is defined as pain associated with a primary site in a person's low back, of musculoskeletal origin and emanating from the lumbar spine. It may include leg pain and/or pain in other areas of the spine. The pain has been present for at least six weeks and it may resolve partially or fully but may often recur (Croft 1988,[2] Hestabaek 2003,[3, 4] Burton 2004[5]).

The GDG considers that 'persistent' describes recurring pain of this nature more precisely than the word 'chronic' which is often used.

These guidelines include people aged between 18 and 65 years with:

- non-specific LBP
- pain lasting for six weeks or more.

People may also have:

- leg pain of spinal origin
- pain associated with other areas of the spine.

These guidelines exclude people with:

- Serious pathology or red flags (section 3.4)
- Osteoporosis
- Pregnancy
- Spondylolisthesis
- A history of spinal surgery
- Radicular pain (i.e., arising from nerve root compromise) (added 18th May 2005).

1.2 The main clinical question

These guidelines focus on a broad clinical question:

Is exercise more effective in terms of improving the health status of people with persistent LBP than no active intervention?

Types of exercise are: mobilising, strengthening, aerobic, general, core stability, hydrotherapy and McKenzie. Six aspects are considered (section 2.5) in relation to effective intervention, these are: reducing pain, improving function, improving psychological status, enabling return to work, cost-effectiveness, and safety. No active intervention is defined as one or more of the following: general practitioner care, a non-physical therapy intervention or a sham intervention.

The literature found compares exercise with non-physiotherapy interventions, other physiotherapy interventions and other exercises (section 4). It was necessary to use these comparisons as the basis

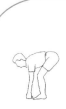

for teasing out whether exercise is more effective than no active intervention. **The GDG found that evidence did not exist to suggest the superiority of one form of exercise over another and saw no benefit in pursuing this question.**

1.3   Objectives

These guidelines focus on exercise as an intervention used by physiotherapists for people with persistent LBP in the UK. The objectives were to develop guidelines that will:

- Assess the quality of the research evidence available
- Make recommendations for future research
- Make treatment recommendations based on the best available evidence
- Improve the quality of patient care by emphasising the best treatment options
- Be user-friendly and practical
- Encourage physiotherapists to engage with reflective practice through reading and applying these guidelines
- Lead to a more consistent approach to the treatment of persistent LBP across the UK (although individual needs and preferences will vary)
- Be accessible for people with persistent LBP
- Enable people with persistent LBP to take a more active role in their treatment where they wish to do so.

1.4   The contribution of these guidelines

Many guidelines making recommendations for people with LBP have already been published but most of these focus on people with acute LBP. These guidelines add substantially to the body of knowledge by focusing on people with persistent LBP by:

- providing a level of detail about exercise, which is likely to be a major component of physiotherapy intervention for people with persistent LBP
- critically appraising the research evidence to indicate the *larger* (section 2.6.5), *higher* methodological quality randomised controlled trials (RCTs) (section 2.6.3), with sufficient data analysis to demonstrate the effectiveness of a particular form of exercise (section 2.6.4)
- addressing the gaps in research evidence with consensus evidence from a group of experts in physiotherapy for people with persistent LBP, from across the UK, and including a patient representative.

Thus these guidelines are based on sound scientific knowledge and expert opinion. They provide a highly practical tool for both clinicians and people with persistent LBP.

1.5   Target users

The authors intend these guidelines to be of particular use to:

- Physiotherapists of all grades who work with people with persistent LBP
- Other professionals involved in the treatment of persistent LBP e.g., general practitioners, occupational therapists and psychologists
- Educational establishments particularly those with an interest in physiotherapy

• People with persistent LBP.

These guidelines were developed in the UK, primarily for use in the UK. Nevertheless the research evidence base is international and the GDG suggest that these guidelines may be applicable outside the UK.

1.6 Epidemiology of persistent LBP

The authors of the European guidelines for the management of chronic non-specific LBP[6] summarise the epidemiology of back pain as follows:
• The lifetime prevalence of LBP is up to 84%

• After an initial episode of LBP, 44-78% of people experience a relapse of pain and 26-37% relapse in terms of absence from work

• Best estimates suggest the prevalence of chronic (persisting for at least 12 weeks), non-specific LBP is approximately 23% and that 11-12% of the population are disabled by LBP

• Specific causes of back pain are uncommon i.e., less than 15% of all back pain.

Persistent LBP is extremely prevalent in our population and the result is that a large proportion of physiotherapists' time is spent in assessing, treating and advising people with this condition.

In 2004 back pain in the UK accounted for:
• 4% of all general practitioner consultations

• 5% of all National Health Service (NHS) specialist referrals

• 13.5% of all UK incapacity benefits.

But receives less than 1.8% of total NHS spending. The best possible care is often not provided and limited and expensive resources are wasted. [7] These guidelines give recommendations for the best possible use of exercise as a physiotherapy intervention for people with persistent LBP.

Human beings have had back pain throughout recorded history; it is no more severe or common than it has always been. However the disability arising from LBP has increased. This can be attributed to social changes from the 1950s to the mid 1990s (i.e., increases in chronic disability, sickness certification and social security benefits), and it is these factors that have changed people's experience and not the pathology or prevalence of back pain.[7] There is an indication of recent reversal of these social trends in some countries.[7]

Nevertheless the course of back pain is variable and it does not always resolve:
• A prospective study indicated that 90% of people with LBP in primary care stop consulting health care practitioners within three months; however most will still be experiencing low back pain and related disability one year after consultation[2]

• A prospective study concluded that LBP should not be considered transient and therefore neglected, since the condition is rarely self-limiting, rather it presents with periodic attacks and temporary remissions[3]

• A review of 36 studies found that LBP does not resolve itself when ignored[4]

• Many people seeking manipulative care for LBP tended to have high levels of recurrence and sought care over at least four years. Because psychosocial factors at presentation exert a long-term influence, they need to be considered by physical therapists.[5]

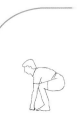

1.7 Terminology

The term 'person with persistent LBP' has been used throughout this document. However there are instances where the word 'patient' was more appropriate and therefore used e.g., patient representative, patient partnership, patient assessment, patient care or patient preference.

1.8 Conflicts of interest

None were declared.

GDG members were authors of papers referred to in these guidelines, which is a reflection that GDG members are experts in this field and was not considered a conflict of interest.

2   Methods

Guidelines are a series of systematically constructed statements devised to assist practitioners with clinical decisions.[8] This section outlines the methods used to develop these guidelines.

2.1   An outline of guideline development methods

A summary of the process for developing clinical guidelines is given below and is adapted from the Scottish Intercollegiate Guidelines Network (SIGN)[9] (figure 2.1).

Figure 2.1 The guideline development process

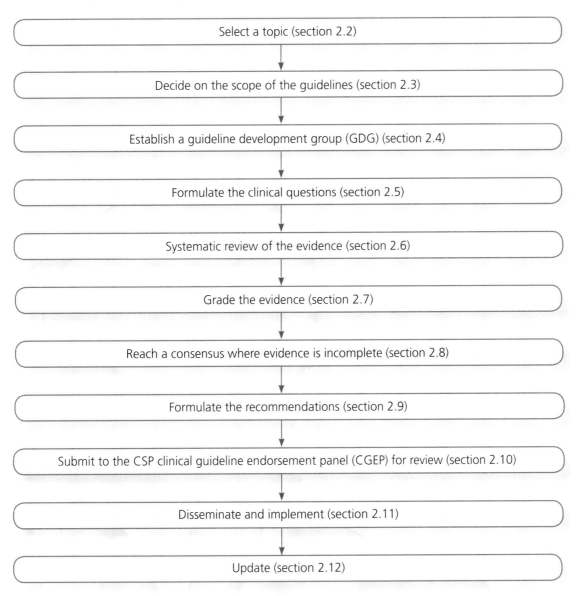

Select a topic (section 2.2)

Decide on the scope of the guidelines (section 2.3)

Establish a guideline development group (GDG) (section 2.4)

Formulate the clinical questions (section 2.5)

Systematic review of the evidence (section 2.6)

Grade the evidence (section 2.7)

Reach a consensus where evidence is incomplete (section 2.8)

Formulate the recommendations (section 2.9)

Submit to the CSP clinical guideline endorsement panel (CGEP) for review (section 2.10)

Disseminate and implement (section 2.11)

Update (section 2.12)

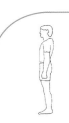

2.2 Selecting the topic

In 2002 the CSP consulted its membership on priority areas for clinical guidelines and persistent LBP was recognised as a major topic.[1]

2.3 Deciding on the scope of the guidelines

The scope of this series of guidelines was decided at a workshop in April 2003. Persistent LBP was defined, the whole range of physiotherapy interventions was included, and exclusion criteria were agreed (appendix A). At a later stage, as a large volume of literature in this field was found, a pragmatic decision was made to divide the project into manageable parts to publish as separate documents. Hence this part focuses on exercise and the second part focuses on manual therapy.

2.4 Establishing a guideline development group (GDG)

A GDG was selected to represent wide ranging expertise including physiotherapists from throughout the UK and from a range of clinical interest groups, academics, patients, policy makers, systematic reviewers and experienced guideline developers (appendix B). The membership of the GDG was not static throughout development of these guidelines, some members stepped down and additional experts were recruited to ensure that the group continued to represent broad thinking.

The representative for the patients' perspective ensured that user perspectives and priorities were high on the agenda. The GDG was facilitated by CSP officers, in particular Dries Hettinga, Katherine Deane and Jo Jordan who reviewed the literature and Anne Jackson who managed the project. Chris Mercer chaired the group.

2.5 Formulating the clinical questions

The scoping process led to the broad clinical question for this part:

Is exercise more effective in terms of improving the health status of people with persistent LBP than no active intervention?

Taking note of the six aspects (see section 1.2) of an effective intervention considered in these guidelines the question was refined to:

Is exercise more effective than no active intervention in reducing pain, improving function and psychological status, and enabling return to work for people aged 18 to 65 years? In addition, is exercise cost effective and safe?

Thus the GDG sought to answer the following six component questions:
- Is exercise more effective than no active intervention in **reducing pain** for people with persistent LBP?

- Is exercise more effective than no active intervention in **improving function** for people with persistent LBP?

- Is exercise more effective than no intervention in **improving psychological status** for people with persistent LBP?

- Is exercise more effective than no active intervention in **enabling return to work** for people with persistent LBP?

- Is exercise a **cost-effective** intervention for people with persistent LBP?

- Is exercise a **safe** therapy for people with persistent LBP?

The first three questions were tackled most effectively owing to the substantive amount of literature in these areas.

2.6 Systematic review

The GDG aimed to find the best available evidence and thus limited the search to RCTs and where this was not available, expert opinion i.e., consensus was used. In terms of the project as a whole, this decision made developing these guidelines a manageable task.

2.6.1 The searches

A large amount of literature relates to LBP and a pragmatic approach identified relevant systematic reviews and RCTs as follows:

- The literature was searched from 1966 to June 2003 (appendix C) for systematic reviews of exercise for people with chronic LBP. This was the main source of RCTs. However these systematic reviews did not completely cover the scope of these guidelines making it necessary to search for additional RCTs

- An extensive literature search of Medline, EMBASE, CINAHL, AMED, PEDro, The Cochrane Library, Sports Discus and the CSP library literature identified RCTs published from 2003 to June 2005 (appendix C)

- The European guidelines for the management of chronic non-specific LBP were used to identify RCTs[6]

- GDG members supplied additional RCTs from personal files.

The references for the studies were imported into bibliographic software (Endnote, version 5) and duplicates eliminated. Titles and abstracts were scanned for RCTs relevant to this review. Full text paper copies of relevant RCTs were obtained for the reviewers.

2.6.2 Inclusion and exclusion criteria

Inclusion criteria for systematic reviews. Papers which:

- Include participants with chronic (defined as persistent here i.e., of six weeks or more duration) non-specific LBP

- Consider exercise as a physiotherapy intervention for persistent LBP

- Compare exercise with no treatment or a placebo or sham procedure, or with other physiotherapy interventions including another type of exercise

- Used mainly RCTs as their data

- Include adult study participants only (aged 18 to 65 years)

- Are written in English.

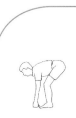

Inclusion criteria for RCTs. Papers which:

- Include participants with chronic (defined as persistent here i.e., of six weeks or more duration) non-specific LBP

- Consider exercise as a physiotherapy intervention for persistent LBP

- Compare exercise with no treatment or a placebo or sham procedure, or with other physiotherapy interventions including another type of exercise

- Include adult participants only (aged 18 to 65 years)

- Are written in English.

Exclusion criteria for RCTs. Papers which include:

- Less than 15 participants in each treatment arm and scores two or less out of 10 on the adapted van Tulder Quality Scale [10]

- Participants with back pain after surgery or resulting from a specific diagnosis e.g., osteoarthritis or spondylolysthesis

- Studies that compare an intervention A with a combination of A and another intervention B. The GDG considered that such a study would not address the major clinical question (section 1.2) i.e., what is the effect of intervention A compared with no active intervention. Results for combinations of interventions would not be straightforward.

2.6.3   Assessment of methodological quality

The GDG chose to use an assessment scale to indicate the quality of RCTs in these guidelines. Readers are advised to consult the evidence tables (appendix D) and, in areas of particular interest, the full paper in order to fully appreciate the critical appraisal process.

The scale chosen was the adapted from the van Tulder Quality Scale[10] which is preferred by the Cochrane Back Review Group. It should be noted that an update of this scale has been published since this systematic review started.[11]

For all papers the quality assessment was carried out twice as indicated below.
The Cochrane systematic reviews by:

- the Cochrane reviewers

- this GDG.

RCTs included in the European guidelines[6] by:

- the European GDG

- this GDG.

Other systematic reviews and other RCTs by:

- two of this GDG's reviewers using the adapted van Tulder Quality Scale. [10]

Evidence tables were developed for each systematic review and RCT and the quality scores were added (appendix D). These tables were used as the basis for the written review (section 4).

This systematic review includes 31 studies, and GDG consensus suggested that it would be useful to highlight those that scored more highly on the adapted van Tulder Quality Scale. This was achieved by selecting ten criteria from the scale (appendix D, table 2), which focused on methodological quality. However, as research and critical appraisal methods are refined, the GDG suggest that this approach may be revised when these guidelines are updated. At the same time, readers are advised that it is important to be up-to-date with critical appraisal methods and consider the methodological quality of studies when considering the reliability of conclusions.

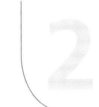

For these guidelines the GDG made a pragmatic decision to make a distinction between RCTs of:

- *higher* methodological quality (i.e., those scoring 5 out of 10, or above or 50% or more) on the adapted van Tulder Quality Scale

- *lower* methodological quality (i.e., those scoring less than 5 out of 10, or less than 50%) on the adapted van Tulder Quality Scale.

2.6.4 Assessment of statistical quality of RCT

As has been stressed (section 1.2) these guidelines focus on the major clinical question:

Is exercise more effective for improving the health status of people with persistent LBP than no active intervention?

RCTs were capable of addressing this question where they compared the differences **between**:
- the effectiveness of one exercise intervention and

- an alternative intervention, or control.

However the review found that a number of RCTs concentrated on **within** group comparisons which are based on two assumptions i.e., that:
- pre-intervention scores are equal in both groups

- LBP, without treatment, does not change over time.

However pre-intervention scores in different groups are not necessarily equal and despite the persistent nature of LBP (section 1.6) there is a suggestion that it may naturally reduce over time.[7] Thus change over time, within any particular group, was discarded as evidence of the effectiveness of any intervention.

The evidence tables display change over time for each intervention group of each trial for each outcome (pain, function, psychological status, return to work and cost) (appendix D, tables 3a-3e). In each case the difference **between** the intervention groups and a control group (or alternative intervention group) is calculated. In the majority of cases original articles have indicated where this difference in change was statistically significant. Nevertheless a number of the trials, in particular older trials, do not report on statistical significance of this difference in change and results of these trials are described as **'inconclusive due to insufficient statistical analysis'** in the text (section 4).

Furthermore the evidence tables (appendix D, tables 3c–3e) express the difference in change **between** the intervention group and a control group (or alternative intervention group) as a percentage of baseline value. These figures are not given in the text to keep the messages to readers as clear as possible.

2.6.5 Assessment of RCT size

Ideally RCTs should include a power calculation to indicate the extent to which the sample size is adequate to demonstrate a difference between comparison groups. This calculation is the preferred way of assessing whether the sample size is adequate. It is normally expected that power is at least 80% and it is based on knowledge of the effect size of the primary outcome measure. The GDG found that only a small minority of included trials had performed a power calculation and it was not feasible for the GDG to carry out this calculation retrospectively.

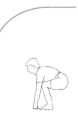

2

In addition, differences between comparison groups may be a result of chance and this is particularly likely where groups are small. To be confident of detecting a real difference clinical trials need to include large numbers of participants.[12] This is particularly the case for studies of people with persistent LBP (which is an unspecific diagnosis) because there is likely to be considerable variability in intervention groups and this means that large comparison group are needed to detect a real difference.

Consequently the GDG made a pragmatic decision to describe the sample size of a trial rather than the power of the trial in this review. By GDG consensus RCTs were defined as:
- *larger* where there were 40 or more participants in the intervention group
- *smaller* where there were less than 40 participants in the intervention group.

Readers should note, in particular, that the acceptability of an intervention group of 40 was chosen arbitrarily and pragmatically, it was not based on theory. As *higher* methodological studies become the norm in physiotherapy the GDG expect that power calculations will be used to assess trials and sample size will thus not be an issue.

Following usual tradition the total number of participants in a RCT is given (section 4). Hence a trial with more than 100 participants may be defined as *smaller* if it has three or more intervention groups e.g., Hemmila's trial (1997 and 2002)[13, 14] (n=132) compares three groups.

2.7 Grading the evidence

An evidence summary is given at the end of each section of the evidence review with an indication of the level of evidence. The levels of evidence used are those recommended in the CSP Information Paper 'Guidance for Developing Clinical Guidelines' (Table 2.1).[15]

Table 2.1 Levels of Evidence, adapted from National Institute for Clinical Excellence (NICE)[16]

Level	Type of evidence
Ia	Evidence obtained from a systematic review of RCTs
Ib	Evidence obtained from at least one RCT
IIa	Evidence obtained from at least one well-designed controlled clinical trial without randomisation or a poor quality RCT.
IIb	Evidence obtained from at least one other type of well-designed quasi-experimental study
III	Evidence obtained from well-designed non-experimental descriptive studies, such as comparative studies, correlation studies and case studies
IV	Evidence obtained from expert committee reports or opinions and/or clinical experience of respected authorities e.g., from the nominal consensus process

To make the literature review a manageable task, the GDG limited their search to systematic reviews and RCTs. No systematic reviews that related directly to the main clinical question (section 1.2) were found.

Findings of an RCT were considered as level **Ib** research evidence if the RCT was:
- of *higher* methodological quality i.e., a score of 5/10 or more on the adapted van Tulder Quality Scale
- of robust statistical quality i.e., a comparison could be made between the effectiveness of an exercise intervention and the effectiveness of a control or alternative intervention
- *larger* i.e., more than 40 participants per treatment arm.

Where RCTs failed to meet one or more of these standards then the findings are described in the text but are not assigned a level of evidence because the GDG considered this evidence unreliable as the basis of a recommendation. However this evidence was used during consensus; the nominal group (section 2.8.2) were encouraged to use the systematic review in order to base their voting on available evidence in addition to experience.

All the evidence found in this review was graded as either **Ib** or **IV**.

2.8 Reaching a consensus where evidence is incomplete

2.8.1 The need for expert consensus

Where the research evidence was either incomplete or inconsistent then consensus evidence was sought for each combination of:

- the three of the clinical questions judged to be within the expertise of the GDG (i.e., is exercise effective in reducing pain, improving function and improving psychological status for people with persistent LBP?) (section 2.5)

- the eight major types of exercise (mobilising, strengthening, aerobic, unsupervised walking, general, core stability, hydrotherapy and McKenzie) that were found in the literature (defined in section 4.2).

Thus there were a total of 24 questions. Of these, seven were answered by the evidence review and the remaining 17 formed the basis of the consensus questionnaire (appendix E1).

2.8.2 Deciding the consensus methods

Four major methods of reaching consensus were discussed by the GDG. They are summarised below (table 2.2).

Table 2.2 Reaching consensus adapted from Heath Technology Assessment[17]

Consensus Method	Description
Informal methods	The GDG reach consensus at an internal meeting.
The Delphi technique	A reference group completes a questionnaire to give expert opinion. Further rounds of the questionnaire, revealing overall opinion, move the group towards consensus.
The nominal group technique	Discussion within the group followed by voting in an iterative process leads to a group judgement.
A consensus development conference	A representative group is brought together to listen to the evidence before retiring to consider the questions and reach a judgement.

The GDG chose the nominal group technique. The Delphi technique and consensus development conference were judged to be unnecessarily expensive, and informal methods lacked credibility and transparency.

The nominal group technique is described by NICE as efficient in terms of time and effectiveness in obtaining consensus:

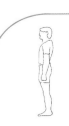

http://www.nice.org.uk/page.aspx?o=308780

and has been used by NICE in the guidelines for preoperative testing (second consultation):
http://www.nice.org.uk/page.aspx?o=36980

To increase the credibility of the consensus process, nine additional experts, chosen for their specialist knowledge in the field of physiotherapy for people with LBP, were asked to join the 14 GDG members who were available to form the nominal group (appendix B) i.e., the nominal group was made up of 23 experts.

NICE suggest using computer technology as a way of communicating during the nominal group technique. The GDG followed this advice to streamline the consensus process and develop the guidelines as efficiently as possible as described below.

The questionnaire contained statements, designed to be direct and unambiguous without giving response cues (appendix E1 and E3). They included a specific population, intervention, comparison and outcome e.g., Reducing pain **(outcome)** for people with persistent LBP **(population)**: mobilising exercises **(intervention)** are more effective than no active intervention **(comparison)** in reducing pain.

2.8.3   Defining consensus

The GDG defined consensus according to the definition used in the CSP's clinical guidelines for the physiotherapy management of whiplash associated disorder[18] (table 2.3).

Table 2.3 Definition of consensus

Percent of respondents	Definition of agreement	Level of evidence
100%	Unanimity	Grade IV
75-99%	Consensus	Grade IV
51-74%	Majority view	No evidence
0-50%	No consensus	No evidence

2.8.4   The consensus process

In a first round of the questionnaire, the nominal group were asked to rate their agreement with 17 statements (agree, neither agree nor disagree, disagree) relating to the 17 questions arising from the literature review. The nominal group were asked to take into account personal opinion, knowledge, experience and the evidence review (section 4). The questionnaire was sent out on 22nd November 2005 and replies were received by 8th December 2005. All communication was by email. Responses of 23 group members were collated on an Excel spreadsheet and the percentage agreements calculated (appendix E4).

Where consensus was achieved (75% or more agreement) then statements were taken out of the questionnaire and became consensus evidence. This was added to the evidence summaries (section 4). Five consensus evidence statements were made after the first round of the questionnaire.

Where consensus was not achieved (less than 75% agreement) a discussion of each question took place on the back pain development site of the interactive CSP (iCSP) (8th December 2005 to 22nd December 2005). The aim was to consider the reasons for different opinions and to work towards consensus. The distribution of responses to each statement on the first round questionnaire was presented with each question. Specific GDG members facilitated the discussions relating to questions where they had particular expertise. The iCSP discussion was also important because it formed the basis of a series of recommendations focused on the application of supervised exercises (section 5.2); an outline of the dialogue is included (appendix E2).

In a second round questionnaire (appendix E3), containing the 12 remaining questions, (indicating group scores and individual scores for the first round) the nominal group was asked to rate agreement with each statement (agree, neither agree nor disagree, disagree). The questionnaire was sent out on 5th January 2006 and all replies were received by 19th January 2006. Again all communication was by email; responses of 23 group members (one of the original group members was sick and another unable to complete the questionnaire in the time frame) were collated on an Excel spreadsheet. The percentage agreement for each question was again calculated (appendix E4).

Each statement that achieved consensus was defined as level **IV** consensus evidence and was added to the evidence summaries 1 to 7 (section 4). The consensus process is summarised (figure 2.2).

2.8.5 Summary of the consensus process

Figure 2.2 Summary of the consensus process

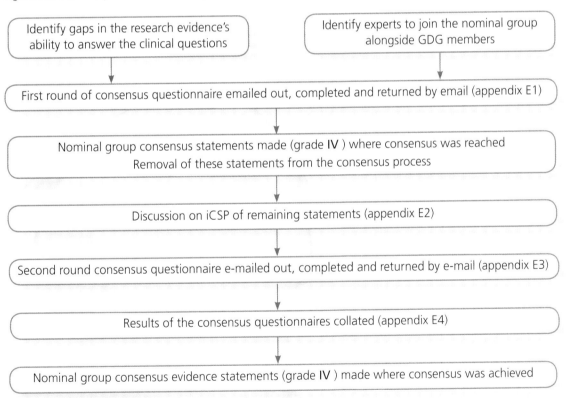

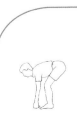

2.9 Formulating the recommendations

Clinical recommendations were formulated from the research evidence and graded according to the type of evidence on which they were based (table 2.4).

Table 2.4 Grading guideline recommendations adapted from NICE[16]

Grade	Evidence
A	At least one RCT of overall higher quality and consistency addressing the specific recommendation (evidence levels Ia and Ib in Table 2.1)
B	Well-conducted clinical studies but not RCTs on the topic of the recommendation (evidence levels IIa, IIb and III in Table 2.1)
C	Evidence from the nominal group technique or other expert committee reports. This indicates that directly applicable clinical studies or higher quality are absent (evidence level IV in Table 2.1)
D	Recommended good practice based on the clinical experience of the GDG

Readers should note that grading the recommendations is a different stage in the process of guideline development to grading the evidence (table 2.1).

The GDG made grade A-C clinical recommendations where there was either:

- research evidence
- or 75% of the nominal group were in agreement, on the first or second round of the questionnaire (table 2.5).

Table 2.5 Summary of the source of the recommendations

Questions about exercise and pain reduction, improved function, psychological status	Number of questions	Recommendations
Research evidence	7	Grade A
Nominal group consensus (75% or more agreement) on the **first** round of the questionnaire	5	Grade C
Nominal group consensus (75% or more agreement) on the **second** round of the questionnaire after discussion	9	Grade C
No consensus after two rounds of the questionnaire and discussion (less than 75% agreement after two rounds of the consensus questionnaire)	3	No recommendations

The GDG met, by telephone conference, on 9th February 2006 to formulate the wording of the recommendations for clinical practice. Several drafts were produced and refining the recommendations continued by email after the meeting. The following information was used to formulate the recommendations:

- Research evidence (section 4) presented according to the eight types of exercise and three outcomes (pain reduction, improvement in function and improvement in psychological status)
- Consensus evidence (section 4) included in the evidence summary boxes
- Previous discussion, in particular details of the iCSP consensus conference (appendix E2)
- GDG expert consensus

- Ongoing email discussion.

The research recommendations were also outlined at the telephone conference above. They were formulated by circulating drafts by email, email discussion (appendix E5) and redrafting until GDG consensus was reached.

2.10 Submission to the CSP clinical guideline endorsement panel (CGEP)

The GDG referred regularly to the AGREE Instrument[19] during the production of these guidelines to ensure they met the AGREE criteria and that the methodology was structured and rigorous.

The GDG submitted some preliminary material to the CGEP for their meeting on 20th October 2005 and met with the CGEP on 15th November 2005 for a discussion of progress. This was extremely useful e.g., in discussing the methods used in the systematic review and consensus process and contributed substantially to the development of the work by the GDG.

The final draft exercise section of guidelines was submitted to the CGEP for their meeting on 17th May 2006 and was endorsed on 27th July 2006. The guidelines were reviewed by:
- two physiotherapy researchers
- a physiotherapy researcher / clinician
- a physiotherapy clinician
- an osteopath.

Following both the reviewers' and the CGEP's comments some amendments were made, for example:
- the GDG reflection on developing these guidelines (section 10) was expanded to include a section on 'comparing these recommendations compared with other findings' (section 10.7)
- the discussion on implementation (section 8) was developed.

2.11 Dissemination and implementation

The CSP will use its news publication *Frontline* and iCSP to increase awareness of the guidelines amongst the membership and beyond. Implementation is considered in more detail later in the document (section 8).

2.12 Updating

It is planned that this section of the CSP guidelines for persistent LBP will be updated in 2011. The CSP procedure for updating will be followed. See also section 9.

The CSP recently completed a review of its guideline development programme and five recommendations were made for the development of physiotherapy evidence based material. This work will be taken forward in 2007 and the process for reviewing material will be incorporated into a new framework. This may affect the date currently identified for updating the guideline.

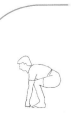

3 Assessment of people with persistent LBP

3.1 Introduction

Readers should note that:

- The GDG do not recommend, or intend to suggest superiority of, any one of the many specialist approaches to assessment of people with persistent LBP. Indeed the group included experts from many fields e.g., the McKenzie and psychosocial approaches. This section is included for completeness and as a general introduction

- It is strongly suggested that where links to other documents are made, readers access the original documents for full details. A systematic review of the literature on assessment was outside the scope of these guidelines and hence this section contains a brief outline with links to further information.

Ideally physiotherapy assessment is holistic and involves the person with persistent LBP in a partnership throughout. The purpose of assessment is to:

- evaluate the pain, functional disability, the psychological impact and the consequences (e.g., on family and work)

- screen for serious pathology (red flags)

- understand people's beliefs and expectations about their problem

- assess barriers to recovery (yellow flags, blue flags and black flags)

- identify impairment (bearing in mind the paucity of evidence suggesting that firm diagnoses can be made)

- negotiate treatment goals with the person with persistent LBP

- negotiate a treatment plan with the person with persistent LBP

- provide specific reassurance and advice about the condition

- decide on outcome measures and collect the relevant data, record and make data available for analysis.

This section summarises some major points relevant to physiotherapy assessment of people with persistent LBP. Much of the detail has been adapted by the GDG from:

- The European guidelines for the management of low back pain (2004)[6] **www.backpaineurope.org**

- The Prodigy guidance for lower back pain (2005)[20] **www.prodigy.nhs.uk/guidance.asp?gt=back+pain+-+lower**

- The Arthritis and Musculoskeletal Alliance (ARMA) standards of care for people with back pain (2004)[21] **www.arma.uk.net/pdfs/bp.pdf#search='arma%20back%20pain%20guidelines**

- The Clinical Standards Advisory Group (CSAG) guidelines[22]

3.2 Evaluating pain and disability

Evaluation of pain and disability is achieved through:

- a patient interview i.e., recording details of people's back pain history and its impact on their lives

- a physical examination i.e., observing, palpating and applying specific tests and people's movement and responses to movement.

3.3   Screening for signs of recovery

GDG consensus suggests two major signs of recovery:

- An indication of return to normal function
- Centralisation i.e., the abolition of distal pain and then spinal pain in response to repeated movements tends to be associated with a good prognosis and occurs in at least 50% of people with persistent LBP[23].

3.4   Screening for serious pathology (red flags)

Red flags are patient responses and findings, on history taking and physical examination, that are associated with possible serious spinal pathology e.g., tumour, infection or fracture. Clinicians need to be aware of the indicators that suggest further investigation by a specialist medical team before physiotherapy intervention is considered. **Note that these guidelines do not make recommendations for people with serious spinal pathology.**

One red flag on its own would not necessarily provide a strong indication of serious pathology; it needs to be considered in the context of the person's history and the findings on examination. A person with more than one red flag is a stronger indicator of serious spinal pathology. It is essential that clinicians remain vigilant to the possibility of serious pathology. The literature suggests a wide variation on what constitutes a red flag; a recent review found 119 different aspects of the patient interview and 44 aspects of the physical examination were cited as red flags, however only 11 of these were consistently rated in more than 50% of papers.[24]

Within the international back pain guidelines there is broad agreement that red flags include:

- Under 20 years old **or** over 55 years old (**and** experiencing first episode of LBP)
- Constant, progressive pain
- Violent trauma
- Previous history of cancer
- Unexplained weight loss
- Systemic steroids
- Intravenous drug use / HIV
- Systemically unwell
- Difficulty with micturition
- Decreased anal tone
- Saddle anaesthesia
- Widespread / progressive neurological signs
- Gait disturbance
- Structural deformity.

Cauda equina syndrome is characterised by the following combination of symptoms and requires immediate referral to the accident and emergency department:

- sphincter (e.g., bladder) disturbance
- sexual dysfunction
- gait disturbance
- saddle anaesthesia.

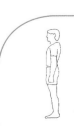

In many cases it is either a combination of factors, or the context of a patient's experience, that leads a clinician to suspect serious spinal pathology. To identify these signs and symptoms it is essential that physiotherapists practising spinal assessments keep abreast of the debate in the literature.

Night time pain has been considered to be a red flag but a recent study of 482 people attending a back pain triage clinic found that 90 of these people had night pain but none had serious pathology.[25] Thus the GDG have not included night pain as a red flag.

Where red flags are detected people may need further investigations e.g.,

- radiography (plain x-rays)
- computed tomography (CT) which uses x-rays to generate cross-sectional spinal images
- magnetic resonance imaging (MRI) which may be most useful for people with radicular symptoms, or for those in whom there is an indication of discitis or neoplasm[6]
- blood tests
- nerve conduction tests.

3.5 Screening for indicators of risk of an ongoing condition (yellow, blue, black flags)

Physiotherapists need to understand people's beliefs and expectations about their pain and they can do this by screening for risk factors of pain related disability. This process encourages holistic intervention tailored to each individual. These psychosocial barriers to recovery, also known as yellow flags, need to be understood and they can be addressed during treatment. They include:

- belief that pain and activity are harmful
- sickness behaviours such as extended rest
- social withdrawal
- emotional problems such as low or negative mood, depression, anxiety, stress
- problems and/or dissatisfaction at work
- disputed or currently unresolved claims for compensation or time off work
- overprotective family or lack of support by family
- inappropriate expectations e.g., of clinician and patient roles in the treatment process, unrealistic expectations of outcome.

People with persistent LBP may have been influenced by terms used by previous medical professionals e.g., that their spine is 'crumbling' or that their discs have 'degenerated and nothing can be done'. Assessment should aim to discover, reassure and correct erroneous beliefs.

A mnemonic has been suggested as an aide-memoire for clinicians to guide them through these topics:
A – attitudes and beliefs about pain
B – behaviours
C – compensation issues
D – diagnosis and treatment issues
E – emotions
F – family
W – work (Waddell 2004[7])

There are other barriers to recovery:

- perceived barriers to return to work (blue flags)
- actual barriers to return to work (black flags) these are usually called organisational obstacles to recovery.[26]

3.6 Identifying functional limitations, goals, plans, reassure

At assessment, physiotherapists identify dysfunction (in the wider sense i.e., physical impairment and level of activity) and, in partnership with the person with persistent LBP, plan the treatment and set realistic treatment goals. Although goals are individual to each person it is likely that they will include one or more of the following:

- reduce pain
- improve ability to function and alleviate disability
- teach suitable coping strategies
- teach strategies to prevent recurrence and the development of chronicity
- increase knowledge and understanding of symptoms.

Taking into account patient preferences, a treatment plan is devised to achieve the agreed goals. People with persistent LBP need to be reassured by a carefully worded and non-threatening explanation about their back pain and engaged in discussion about how the dysfunction can be managed and the expected prognosis. All this needs to be in a language that the person with persistent LBP can understand. Recent evidence suggests that where patients engage with decisions and managing their own health care the service is appropriate and cost effective and outcomes are improved.[27]

3.7 Outcome measures

The core standards of physiotherapy practice (standard 10.4) indicate that outcomes needs to be measured at the beginning and end of treatment to assess its impact.[28] Often people with persistent LBP complete a questionnaire to measure outcomes prior to treatment, immediately post-treatment and, where possible, at a specified time post-treatment (e.g., six months later). It may be recommended that, to reduce bias, outcome questionnaires are not completed in front of physiotherapists, friends or family. Nevertheless measures vary and specific instructions must be followed to ensure validity and reliability.

There are many outcome measures in existence and choice of measure involves consideration of the setting in which it is used, and the validity, reliability and practicality of the measure. There are many variables and the GDG is not in a position to recommend particular measures to use. Nevertheless, the GDG have identified some outcome measures, believed to be in common use, and some links to sources of further information. The measures are organised according to whether they focus on changes in pain, function or psychological status but it should be emphasised that many measures consider more than one of these dimensions.

Pain

- The visual analogue scale (VAS) **www.painsociety.org/pain_scales.html** is frequently used but the GDG suggest that a numerical rating scale (NRS) may be preferred by patients[29] **http://www.csp.org.uk/director/effectivepractice/outcomemeasures/database.cfm?item_id=57 0119BFE46871734E078C4CEB1F66D5**
- The Quebec back pain disability scale[30]
- The Aberdeen low back pain scale[31] which also measures some aspects of function.

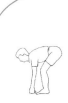

27

Function

- Disability e.g., the Roland-Morris disability questionnaire (RDQ)[32]
- The Oswestry disability index (ODI)[33]
- Quality of life e.g., the short form 36 health survey questionnaire (SF-36).[34] For further information see: www.sf-36.com
- The World Health Organisation Disability Assessment Schedule II (WHO DAS II).[35] For further information see: http://www.who.int/icidh/whodas/.

Psychological status

- Self-efficacy e.g., the chronic pain self-efficacy scale (CPSS)[36]
- Somatic and depressive symptoms e.g., the distress risk assessment method (DRAM)[37]
- The fear avoidance beliefs questionnaire[38]
- The back beliefs questionnaire, designed to measure beliefs about the inevitable consequences of future life with low back problems[39]
- Tampa scale for Kinesiophobia[40]
- Depression, anxiety and positive outlook scale (DAPOS).[41] For further information see: www.dapos.org.

Some further points about outcome measures:

- The VAS, RDQ and ODI may be currently the most commonly used outcome measures in physiotherapy departments in the UK
- Readers interested in research in this area should refer to the outcome measures recommended for clinical trials of chronic pain[29] (See also section 6.3)
- Readers should access the following document that discusses outcome measures for LBP related functional limitations:

  http://www.csp.org.uk/search/result.cfm?item_ID=74C872D6B0AE9DA17B41E7FEB586B866& module=publications&cat=5C62E0AB93918823FDB3B0CFA6654A6B

- Standardisation of outcome measures used would facilitate the comparison of results across studies.[42]

4 Exercise

4.1 Introduction

A total of 31 RCTs considering exercise as an intervention used by physiotherapists for people with persistent LBP were found. This section defines each type of exercise included i.e., mobilising, strengthening, aerobic, general, core stability, hydrotherapy, McKenzie and coordination. Following this, the effectiveness of each type of exercise is compared with:

- Non-physiotherapy or control interventions e.g., placebo or sham interventions, general practitioner care, 'usual care', no treatment or waiting list controls

- Other physiotherapy intervention e.g., manual therapy, back schools

- Other exercise interventions.

The effects of the interventions are evaluated in both the short-term (less than six months post-intervention) and long-term (six months or more post-intervention).

To give a flavour of the literature as a whole, some details of less robust studies are given. However all level **Ib** evidence, presented in the research evidence summary boxes, is derived only from *larger, higher* methodological quality trials with robust statistical analysis. The RCTs are defined as follows (table 4.1):

Table 4.1 Assessing the RCTs

Criteria	Categories	Definition of RCT
Number of participants per group investigated	Less than 40	*Smaller*
	More than or equal to 40	*Larger*
Quality score	Less than 5/10	*Lower* methodological quality
	More than or equal to 5/10	*Higher* methodological quality
Additional improvement in one group, compared with another group, calculated?	No	Results are inconclusive due to insufficient statistical analysis
	Yes	Robust statistics

It should be noted that many trials allocate participants to three or more groups thus the total number of participants given for each RCT, does not necessarily indicate a *smaller* or *larger* trial. However where trials are *larger* and of *higher* quality this is emphasised in the text. Where results are inconclusive due to insufficient statistical analysis this is also emphasised.

To indicate methodological quality of trials a score out of 10 is given to each trial. This is the sum of the 10 items that score positively for internal validity on the adapted van Tulder Quality Scale[10] (appendix D, table 2). Readers are reminded that these quality scores:

- are a simplification of reality

- relate to the above ten items only

- should be considered a representation of the methodological quality of trials i.e., not their actual quality.

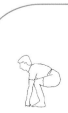

Figure 4.1 Number of trials achieving each quality score

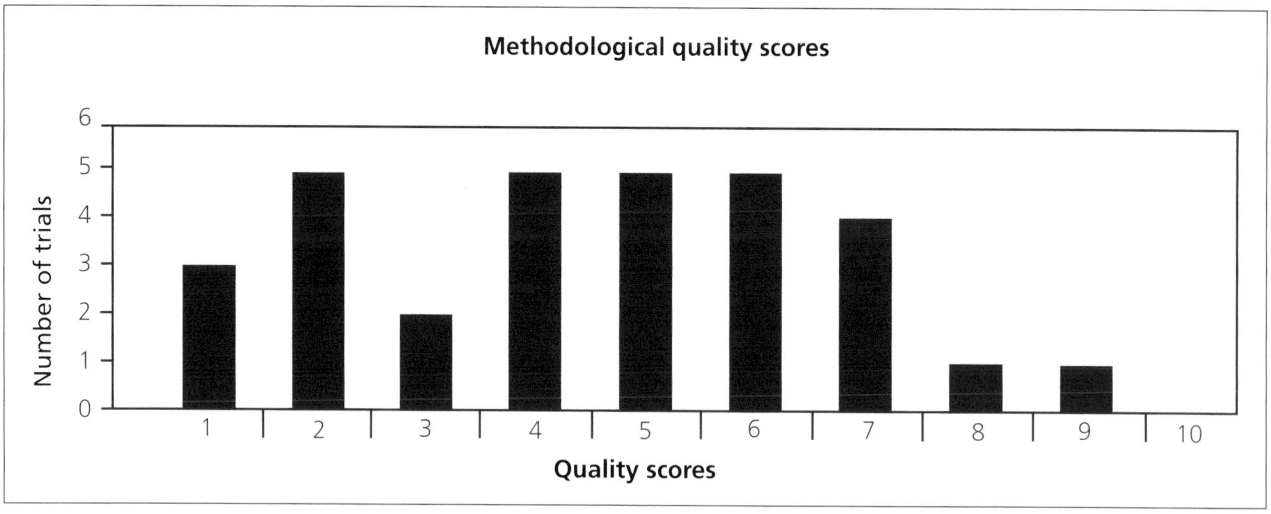

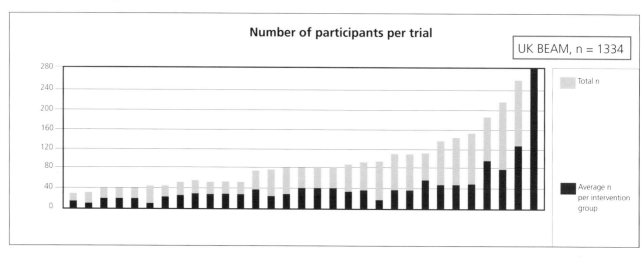

The median methodological quality score is 5 (figure 4.1) but in general the scores of the RCTs show great variation. Fifteen of the 31 RCTs had a score lower than 5 (i.e., they are *lower* in quality) and eight of these have only a score of one or two.

The size of the trials also greatly varies, as is seen in the graph below (figure 4.2)

Figure 4.2 Summary of size of trials

The median number of participants in the included trials is 41 but many trials have more than two intervention groups, and this greatly reduces the power of the trial. The median size of intervention groups for included trials to 30. The UK BEAM trial is exceptionally large in having 1334 participants in four intervention groups, on the other hand 20 of the 31 RCTs had fewer than 40 participants in each intervention group.

The consensus questions filled the gaps in the literature and the consensus evidence is given in this section after the research evidence in the evidence summary boxes. The level of nominal group consensus agreement is given in words (as defined in table 2.3), and as a percentage, whether agreement was first or second round is stated, and the evidence is graded (i.e., grade **IV** or **not graded**).

4.2   Defining exercise

Exercise is defined by the GDG as physical exertion, with instruction or advice of a physiotherapist, aimed at gaining increased movement of spinal joints, increased strength of spinal muscles, increased general fitness, building core stability and/or reducing symptoms.

These definitions were discussed and written by the GDG, suitable definitions were not found in dictionaries of physiotherapy.

The GDG defined exercise according to the definitions in research papers but recognise that there is overlap e.g., aerobic exercise is likely to influence mobility, strength and coordination.

Mobilising exercises where the aim is to increase people's ability to move:

* flexion mobilising exercises: to gain more forward bend of the spine

* extension mobilising exercises: to gain more backward bend of the spine

* general mobilising exercises: to gain more flexibility of the spine, in all directions.

Strengthening exercises where the aim is to increase people's muscle strength:

* flexion strengthening exercises: to gain more strength of abdominal muscles

* extension strengthening exercises: to gain more strength of muscles around the back of the spine

* general strengthening exercises: to gain increased strength of muscles around the abdomen, spine and the rest of the body.

Aerobic exercises: where the aim is to increase general fitness and a healthy cardiovascular system by exercising at a pace where additional effort is needed by the lungs and heart to meet the demand for oxygen from the skeletal muscles.

Unsupervised walking: where people are simply advised to walk regularly. This is defined by the GDG as an aerobic exercise but is considered separately because it differs from organised aerobic exercise programmes.

General exercises: any combination of mobilising exercises, strengthening exercises, aerobic exercises.

Core stability exercises: where the aim is to improve control of deep trunk stabilising muscles thus to increase the ability of muscles to support normal trunk and limb movement.

Hydrotherapy exercises: where the aim is to gain flexibility of joints, strength of muscles, core stability, general fitness and improved function. They are performed in warm water (32 – 35°Celsius) and use the physical properties of water to enhance the effect of the exercises. The warmth and buoyancy of the water makes exercise possible for people who cannot easily move out of water as a result of pain, stiffness or loss of confidence.

McKenzie exercises: direction specific exercises to treat symptoms of LBP. More specifically this approach is based on the McKenzie method of mechanical diagnosis and therapy, which is a system of assessment and management that uses classification by non-specific mechanical syndromes. Assessment involves the monitoring of symptomatic and mechanical responses during the use of repeated

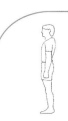

movements and sustained postures. Management involves both direction specific exercises (extension, lateral glide, or flexion) and passive mobilisation procedures if required. Direction specific exercises are clinically determined by abolition, centralisation or decrease in symptoms, increase in range of movement or other suitable responses.

Coordination exercises: work towards achieving harmonious functioning of the body's organs and parts. Through exercise the brain's motor apparatus is encouraged to use groups of muscles, simultaneously, to perform useful functional tasks.

4.3 Mobilising exercises

Flexion mobilising exercises, extension mobilising exercises and general mobilising exercises are included.

4.3.1 Mobilising exercises versus non-physiotherapy interventions

No RCTs were identified.

4.3.2 Mobilising exercises versus other physiotherapy interventions

No RCTs were identified.

4.3.3 Mobilising exercises versus other exercises

Two RCTs were found: Tritilanunt 2001[43] and Elnagger 1991[44].

Tritilanunt's[43] trial (n=72) was of *higher* methodological quality (6/10) and reported that mobilising exercises, compared with an aerobic exercises, were less effective in reducing pain (short-term).

Elnagger's[44] (n=56) **higher** methodological quality trial (5/10) found flexion mobilising exercises and extension mobilising exercises were similarly effective in reducing pain (short-term).

Evidence summary 1: Mobilising exercises

Research evidence

There is no *larger, higher* quality RCT, with sufficient statistical analysis to support or refute the use of mobilising exercises rather than:

- non-physiotherapy interventions
- other physiotherapy interventions
- other exercises.

Nominal group consensus

Mobilising exercises may be more effective than no active intervention in:

- improving function (consensus 91%, second round) IV
- reducing pain (consensus 83%, second round) IV
- improving psychological status (consensus 83%, second round) IV

Recommendations: mobilising exercises

Mobilising exercises should be considered when aiming to:
- improve function   C
- reduce pain   C
- improve psychological status   C

4.4   Strengthening exercises

Flexion strengthening exercises, extension strengthening exercises and general strengthening exercises are included.

4.4.1   Strengthening exercises versus non-physiotherapy interventions

Two RCTs were found: Donchin 1990[45] and Martin 1986[46].

A *larger* (n=142) and *higher* methodological quality (5/10) trial by Donchin[45] found that a callisthenics programme (i.e., flexion strengthening exercises), compared with untreated controls, is:
- more effective in reducing pain (long-term).

Martin's[46]. trial (n=36) had less than 15 participants per group and a methodological quality of 1/10, hence it was not considered in this review (section 2.6.2).

4.4.2   Strengthening exercises versus other physiotherapy interventions

Two RCTs were found: Donchin 1990[45] and Manniche 1991[47].

Donchin's[45] *larger* (n=142) and *higher* methodological quality (5/10) trial found that a flexion strengthening exercise programme, compared with a back school, was:
- more effective in reducing pain (long-term).

Manniche's[47] trial (n=105) had a methodological quality of 2/10 and compared general back strengthening programmes (both high intensity and a low intensity programmes) with a specified physiotherapy programme (massage, hot compresses and mild isometric exercises). The high intensity strengthening programme, compared with the physiotherapy programme, was:
- more effective in reducing pain and improving function (short-term)
- similarly effective in reducing pain and improving function (long-term).

The low intensity strengthening programme, compared with the physiotherapy programmes, was:
- similarly effective in pain reduction (short-term and long-term)
- similarly effective in improving function (short-term and long-term).

4.4.3   Strengthening exercises versus other exercises

Six RCTs were found: Petersen 2002,[48] Koumantakis 2005,[49] Rittweger 2002,[50] Helmhout 2004,[51] Manniche 1991,[47] and Martin 1986[46].

Petersen's[48] trial was *larger* (n=260) and *higher* in methodological quality (6/10). An intensive strengthening exercise programme, compared with a McKenzie therapy group, was found to be:

- similarly effective in improving function (immediately after intervention)
- less effective in improving function (short-term)
- similarly effective in improving function (long-term)
- similarly effective in reducing pain (short- and long-term)
- similarly effective in enabling return to work (short- and long-term).

Koumantakis's[49] trial (n=55) was of *higher* methodological quality (7/10) and compared combined exercises (general stabilising and strengthening exercises) with general strengthening exercises. Both groups also received the Back Book[52] containing written advice. Strengthening alone, compared with the combined programme, was:

- more effective in improving function (short-term, 8 weeks post-intervention)
- similarly effective in improving function (short-term, 20 weeks post-intervention)
- similarly effective in improving function (long-term)
- similarly effective in reducing pain (short and long-term)
- similarly effective in improving psychological status (short-term).

Rittweger's[50] trial (n=60) with a methodological quality of 4/10 compared extension strengthening exercises with exercises conducted on a vibrating platform. The programmes were:

- similarly effective in reducing pain (short-term)
- similarly effective in improving function (short- and long-term).

The effects on depression were inconclusive due to insufficient statistical analysis (section 2.6.4).

Helmhout's[51] *larger* trial (n=81) with a methodological quality of 3/10 compared a high intensity strengthening programme with a low intensity strengthening programme. The programmes were:

- similarly effective in improving function (short- and long-term)
- similarly effective in reducing fear of movement (short- and long-term).

Manniche's[47] trial (n=105) with a methodological quality of 2/10 found that a high intensity back strengthening programme, compared to a low intensity back strengthening programme was:

- more effective in reducing pain and improving (short-term)
- similarly effective in reducing pain and improving function (long-term).

Martin's[46] trial (n=36) had less than 15 participants per group and a methodological quality of 1/10, thus it was not considered in this review (section 2.6.2).

Evidence summary 2: Strengthening exercises

Research evidence

Flexion strengthening exercises are:

- more effective than no treatment in reducing pain (long-term) **Ib**
- more effective than back schools in reducing pain (long-term) **Ib.**

(Donchin[45])

Intensive strengthening exercises compared with McKenzie therapy are:

- less effective in improving function (short-term) **Ib**
- similarly effective in improving function (long-term) **Ib**
- similarly effective in reducing pain (short- and long-term) **Ib**
- similarly effective in enabling return to work (short- and long-term) **Ib.**

(Petersen[48])

Nominal group consensus

Strengthening exercises may be more effective than no active intervention in:

- improving psychological status (87% consensus, second round) **IV**
- improving function (80% consensus, first round) **IV.**

Recommendations: strengthening exercises

Strengthening exercises should be considered when aiming to:

- reduce pain .... A
- improve psychological status C
- improve function. C

4.5   Aerobic exercises

This includes walking and general aerobic exercise programmes.

4.5.1   Aerobic exercises versus non-physiotherapy interventions

Two RCTs were found: Turner 1990[53] and Storheim 2003[54].

Storheim's[54] trial (n=93) of *higher* methodological quality (5/10) found that aerobic exercises, compared with general practitioner care, were:

- similarly effective in reducing pain (short-term)
- similarly effective in improving function (short-term)
- more effective in reducing fear avoidance (short-term)
- similarly effective in reducing emotional distress (short-term).

Turner's[53] trial (n=96) with a methodological quality of 4/10 compared aerobic exercises with a waiting list control group but the results were inconclusive due to sufficient statistical analyses (section 2.6.4).

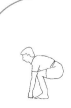

4.5.2 Aerobic exercises versus other physiotherapy interventions

Four RCTs were found: Torstensen 1998,[55] Mannion 1999,[56] Storheim 2003,[54] and Turner 1990[53].

Mannion's[56] trial was *larger* (n=148) and *higher* in methodological quality (9/10). It found that aerobic exercises, compared with physical mixed methods (e.g., combinations of TENS, ultrasound, exercises), were:
- more effective in improving psychological status (short-term)
- similarly effective in improving psychological status (long-term)
- similarly effective in reducing pain (short and long-term)
- similarly effective in improving function (short and long-term).

In Mannion's[56] trial the aerobic exercise programme was structured but in Torstensen's,[55] trial the exercise was unstructured (because it was designed as the control group), participants were simply encouraged to walk for at least an hour a week. In both trials a wide range of interventions were included in the standard physiotherapy group thus there was no standard comparison group.

Torstensen's[55] trial was *larger* (n=208) and *higher* in methodological quality (8/10). It reported that unsupervised aerobic exercise (walking) compared with physical mixed methods (e.g., combinations of TENS, ultrasound, and exercises), was:
- less effective in reducing pain (short and long-term)
- more effective in improving function (short and long-term).

Storheim's[54] trial (n=93) of *higher* methodological quality (5/10) compared an aerobic exercise programme with a cognitive intervention (i.e., about the benefits of both exercise and returning to normal activity). The exercise programme, compared with the cognitive intervention, was:
- similarly effective in reducing pain and improving function (short-term)
- similarly effective in reducing fear avoidance (short-term)
- less effective in improving emotional distress (short-term).

Turner's[53] trial (n=96) had a methodological quality of 4/10. The exercise programme, compared with a behavioural intervention, was:
- similarly effective in reducing pain and improving function (short- and long-term).

4.5.3 Aerobic exercises versus other exercises

Four RCTs were found: Torstensen (1998),[55] Mannion 1999,[56] Tritilanunt 2001,[43] and Johannsen 1995[57].

Mannion's[56] trial was *larger* (n=145) and *higher* in methodological quality (9/10) and compared aerobic exercises with muscle reconditioning (similar to functional restoration and using devices to strengthen various muscle groups). The aerobic programme was:
- similarly effective in reducing pain (short and long-term)
- similarly effective in improving function (short and long-term)
- similarly effective in improving psychological status (short and long-term).

The muscle reconditioning groups exercise included strengthening exercises, a warm up aerobic component, relaxation and stretching. This was defined as general exercise by the GDG (section 4.6). There is research evidence that general exercises are effective in reducing pain and improving function (evidence summary 4). Hence, aerobic exercises must also be effective in terms of both these outcomes.

Torstensen's[55] *larger* (n=208) and *higher* quality trial (8/10) found that aerobic exercise (walking, designed as the control group), compared with medical exercise therapy including strengthening and mobilising exercises, was:

- less effective in reducing pain (short and long-term)
- less effective in improving function (short and long-term).

Tritilanunt's[43] trial (n=72) of *higher* methodological quality (6/10) reported significantly more reduction in pain (short-term) in an aerobic exercises group than for a flexion mobilising group, but no other results were reported.

Johannsen's[57] trial (n=40) was of methodological quality 1/10. A large attrition rate meant that there were less than 15 participants in each group and thus the results of this study are not considered here (section 2.6.2).

Evidence summary 3a: aerobic exercises

Research evidence

Organised aerobic exercises, compared with physical mixed methods, are:
- more effective in improving psychological status (short-term) **Ib**
- similarly effective in improving psychological status (long-term) **Ib**
- similarly effective in reducing pain (short- and long-term) **Ib**
- similarly effective in improving function (short- and long-term) **Ib**.

(Mannion[56])

Organised aerobic exercises, compared with muscle reconditioning exercises, are:
- similarly effective in reducing pain (short- and long-term) **Ib**
- similarly effective in improving function (short- and long-term) **Ib**
- similarly effective in improving psychological status (short- and long-term) **Ib**.

(Mannion[56])

There is no *larger, higher* quality RCT, with sufficient statistical analysis to support or refute the use of aerobic exercises rather than non-physiotherapy interventions.

Nominal group consensus

- Organised aerobic exercises may be more effective than no active intervention in improving psychological status (96% consensus, first round) **IV**.

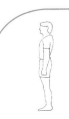

Evidence summary 3b: unsupervised walking

Research evidence

Unsupervised walking, compared with physical mixed methods, is:
- less effective in reducing pain (short- and long-term) **Ib**
- more effective in improving function (short- and long-term) **Ib.**

(Torstensen[55])

Unsupervised walking, compared with general exercises, are:
- less effective in reducing pain (short- and long-term) **Ib**
- less effective in improving function (short- and long-term) **Ib.**

(Torstensen[55])

Nominal group consensus

Unsupervised walking may be more effective than no active intervention in:
- improving psychological status (84% consensus, first round) **IV**
- improving function (76% consensus, first round) **IV**
- reducing pain (74% majority view, second round) **not graded.**

Recommendations: organised aerobic exercises

Organised aerobic exercises should be considered when aiming to:
- reduce pain   A
- improve function   A
- improve psychological status.   C

Recommendations: unsupervised walking

People should be advised of the benefits of unsupervised walking in:
- improving psychological status   C
- improving function.   C

4.6   General exercises

Including combinations of: mobilising, aerobic and strengthening exercises.

4.6.1   General exercises versus non-physiotherapy interventions

Eight RCTs studies were found: Klaber Moffett 1999,[58] Callaghan 1994,[59] Kuukkanen 2000,[60] Snook 1998,[61] Hemmila 1997 and 2002,[13, 14] Martin 1986,[46] Risch 1993,[62] and UK BEAM 2004[63, 64].

Klaber Moffett's[58] trial was *larger* (n=187) and of *higher* methodological quality (7/10). A 'Back to Fitness' programme (aimed at low impact aerobic, and strengthening exercises) was compared with standard general practitioner care. The general exercise programme was:
- more effective in reducing (distressing) pain (long-term)
- similarly effective in reducing (distressing) pain (short-term)

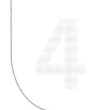

- more effective in improving function (long-term)

- similarly effective in improving function (short-term).

The UK BEAM trial[63, 64] was *larger* (n=1334) and of *higher* methodological quality (6/10). The authors reported that exercise (a Back to Fitness programme based on cognitive behavioural principles) combined with best general practitioner care, compared with best general practitioner care alone, was:

- more effective in reducing pain (short-term)

- more effective in reducing pain (long-term)

- more effective in improving function (short-term)

- more effective in reducing fear avoidance behaviour (short-term)

- similarly effective in improving function (long-term)

- similarly effective in reducing fear avoidance behaviour (long-term).

Hemmila's[13, 14] trial (n=132) of *higher* methodological quality (7/10) compared a general home exercise programme (strengthening and mobilising) with bone setting by traditional folk healers. The exercise programme was:

- more effective in improving function (long-term)

- similarly effective in improving function (short-term)

- similarly effective in reducing sick leave (short- and long-term)

- similarly effective in reducing pain (short-term)

- less effective in reducing pain (long-term).

This RCT was defined as *smaller* because it had three intervention groups and a high attrition rate. Further although bone setting is a physical therapy, it is classified here as a non-physiotherapy intervention because it is outside the scope of usual UK physiotherapy practice. For both these reasons its effectiveness in reducing long-term pain did not lead to a recommendation.

Snook's[61] trial did not investigate the effectiveness of an exercise intervention, rather it described exercise as a sham intervention, and hence it is not considered here. The remaining four trials were *smaller* and *lower* in methodological quality and hence do not add to the evidence (Callaghan,[59] Kuukkanen,[60] Risch,[62] and Martin[46]).

4.6.2 General exercises versus other physiotherapy interventions

Seven RCTs were found: Mannion 1999,[56] Torstensen 1998,[55] UK BEAM 2004,[63, 64] Hemmila 1997 and 2002,[13, 14] Gur 2003,[65] Joussett 2004,[66] and Kankaapaa 1999[67].

Mannion's[56] trial was *larger* (n=148) and *higher* in methodological quality (9/10). It compared:

- general exercises (combined strengthening and mobilizing exercises)

- physical mixed methods (TENS, ultrasound therapy, short wave therapy, heat and cold and some exercises).

The general exercises, in comparison with the physical mixed methods were:

- more effective in improving psychological status (long-term)

- similarly effective (in improving psychological status (short-term)

- similarly effective in reducing pain (short and long-term)

- similarly effective in improving function (short and long-term).

Torstensen's[55] trial was *larger* (n=208) and of *higher* methodological quality (8/10). Medical exercise

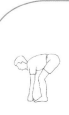

therapy (general mobilising and strengthening exercises) compared to standard physiotherapy interventions (e.g., massage, electrotherapy, traction) was:

- similarly effective in reducing pain (short- and long-term)
- similarly effective in improving function (short- and long-term).

The UK BEAM trial[63, 64] was *larger* (n=1334) and *higher* in methodological quality (6/10). It included groups receiving combined:

- general exercises (a Back to Fitness programme based on cognitive behavioural principles) and best general practitioner care
- manipulation and best general practitioner care.

This trial was designed to assess the additional value of exercise, manipulation, or exercise in combination with manipulation over general practitioner care. Results comparing the effectiveness of the exercise programme versus the effectiveness of the manipulation programme are not presented. Therefore results are inconclusive in terms of this section, the trial did not directly compare exercises with another physiotherapy intervention.

Hemmila's[13, 14] trial (n=132) of *higher* methodological quality (7/10) compared a general exercise programme with a range of mixed interventions (e.g., manual therapy, electrotherapy, thermal therapies, massage and manual traction). The interventions were similarly effective in reducing pain (short- and long-term), improving function (short- and long-term) and reducing sick leave (short- and long-term).

Gur's[65] trial (n=75) of *higher* methodological quality (5/10) compared:

- a general exercise programme (focussing on strengthening and mobilising exercises)
- laser therapy
- laser therapy combined with exercises.

The interventions were equally effective in reducing pain (short-term) and improving function (short-term).

Joussett's[66] trial (n=83) of methodological quality 4/10 compared an active individual therapy programme (home exercises and supervised exercises aimed at flexibility, strengthening and increasing aerobic performance) with a functional restoration programme. The results were inconclusive due to insufficient statistical analysis (section 2.6.4).

The remaining trial by Kankaapaa[67] was *smaller*, of methodological quality 3/10 and did not add to this review.

4.6.3 General exercises versus other exercises

Six RCTs were found: Mannion 1999,[56] Torstensen 1998,[55] Yozbatiran 2004,[68] Reilly 1989,[69] Callaghan 1994,[59] and Martin 1986[46].

Mannion's[56] trial was *larger* (n=148) and *higher* in methodological quality (9/10). A general strengthening and mobilising exercises programme, compared with an aerobic exercise programme, was:

- similarly effective in reducing pain (short- and long-term)
- similarly effective in improving function (short- and long-term)
- similarly effective in improving psychological status (short- and long-term).

Torstensen's[55] trial was *larger* (n=208) and of *higher* methodological quality (8/10). Medical exercise therapy (strengthening and mobilising exercises) using specially designed exercise equipment compared with the aerobic exercises (walking) was:

- more effective in reducing pain (short-term)
- more effective in reducing pain (long-term)
- more effective in improving function (short-term)
- more effective in reducing pain (long-term).

Yozbatiran's[68] trial (n=30) was *higher* in methodological quality (5/10) and compared a general exercise programme (warm-up, stretching, 15 progressive exercises and light aerobic exercises) with hydrotherapy (defined as the same exercises performed in water). The results were inconclusive due to insufficient statistical analysis (section 2.6.4) but there was similar pain reduction in both groups.

The remaining three trials (Reilly,[69] Callaghan,[59] and Martin[46]) were not of sufficient size and quality to add to the evidence.

Evidence summary 4: General exercises

Research evidence

A general exercise programme, compared with standard general practitioner care, is:
- more effective in reducing (distressing) pain (long-term) **Ib**
- more effective in improving function (long-term) **Ib**
- similarly effective in reducing (distressing) pain (short-term) **Ib**
- similarly effective in improving function (short-term) **Ib**.

(Klaber Moffett[58])

General exercises, compared with standard physical mixed methods, are:
- similarly effective in reducing pain (short- and long-term) **Ib**
- similarly effective in improving function (short- and long-term) **Ib**.

(Torstensen[55])

General exercise, compared with best general practitioner care, is:
- more effective in reducing pain (short- and long-term) **Ib**
- more effective in improving function (short-term) **Ib**
- more effective in improving fear avoidance behaviour (short-term) **Ib**
- similarly effective in improving function (long-term) **Ib**
- similarly effective in improving fear avoidance behaviour (long-term) **Ib**.

(UK BEAM[63, 64])

General exercises compared with physical mixed methods, are:
- more effective in improving psychological status (long-term) **Ib**
- similarly effective in improving psychological status (short-term) **Ib**
- similarly effective in reducing pain (short- and long-term) **Ib**
- similarly effective in improving function (short- and long-term) **Ib**.

(Mannion[56])

A general exercise programme, compared with aerobic exercise (walking), is:
- more effective in reducing pain (short and long-term) **Ib**
- more effective in improving function (short and long-term) **Ib**.

(Torstensen[55])

> ### Evidence summary 4: General exercises
>
> A general exercise programme, compared with an aerobic exercise programme, is:
> - similarly effective in reducing pain (short- and long-term) **Ib**
> - similarly effective in improving function (short- and long-term) **Ib**
> - similarly effective in improving psychological status (short- and long-term) **Ib**.
>
> (Mannion[56])
>
> **Nominal group consensus**
> - General exercises may be more effective than no active intervention in improving psychological status (88% consensus, first round) **IV**

> ### Recommendations: general exercise
>
> General exercises should be considered when aiming to:
> - reduce pain   **A**
> - improve function   **A**
> - improve psychological status.   **C**

4.7 Core stability exercises

Exercises to improve control of the trunk muscles and to increase the ability of muscles to support normal trunk and limb movement are included.

4.7.1 Core stability exercises versus non-physiotherapy interventions

One RCTs was found: Shaughnessy 2004[70].

Shaughnessy's[70] trial (n=41) with a methodological quality of 2/10 found that a lumbar core stabilisation programme compared with a 'no treatment' group, was more effective in improving function (short-term).

4.7.2 Core stability exercises versus other physiotherapy interventions

One RCT was found: Rasmussen-Bar 2003[71].

Rasmussen-Bar's[71] trial (n=47) had a methodological quality of 2/10. Core stability exercises were compared with manual treatment. The interventions were similarly effective in reducing pain (short and long-term) and in improving function (short- and long-term).

4.7.3 Core stability exercises versus other exercises

One RCT was found: Koumantakis 2005[49].

Koumantakis's[49] trial (n=55) was of *higher* methodological quality (7/10). A stabilisation enhanced general exercise programme, in comparison with a general strengthening exercise programme, was:
- less effective in improving function (short-term, 8 weeks post-intervention)

42

- similarly effective in improving function (short-term, 20 weeks post-intervention)
- similarly effective in improving function (long-term)
- similarly effective in reducing pain (short-term and long-term)
- similarly effective in improving psychological status (short-term).

Evidence summary 5: Core stability exercises

Research evidence

There is no *larger, higher* quality RCT, with sufficient statistical analysis to support or refute the use of core stability exercises rather than:
- non-physiotherapy interventions
- other physiotherapy interventions
- other exercises.

Nominal group consensus

Core stability exercises may be more effective than no active intervention in:
- improving function (consensus 83%, second round) **IV**
- reducing pain (majority view 74%, second round) **not graded**
- improving psychological status (consensus 61%, second round) **not graded.**

Recommendations: core stability exercises

Core stability exercises should be considered when aiming to:
- improve function.   C

4.8   Hydrotherapy

Including exercises performed in warm water (32 – 35 Celsius) using the properties of water to enhance the effect of the exercises.

4.8.1   Hydrotherapy versus non-physiotherapy interventions

One RCT was found: McIlveen (1998)[72].

McIlveen's[72] larger (n=109) and *higher* methodological trial (6/10) trial indicated that in the hydrotherapy group, compared with waiting list controls:
- statistically significantly more participants reported improved function (short-term)
- there was no statistically significant differences in terms of participants whose pain reduced (short-term).

No long-term outcomes were reported.

4.8.2   Hydrotherapy versus other physiotherapy interventions

No RCTs comparing hydrotherapy with other physiotherapy interventions were found.

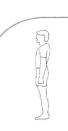

4.8.3 Hydrotherapy versus other exercises

No RCTs comparing hydrotherapy with other exercises were found.

Evidence summary 6: Hydrotherapy

Research evidence

Hydrotherapy exercises, compared with waiting list controls are:
- more effective in improving function (short-term) **Ib**
- similarly effective in reducing pain (short-term) **Ib.**

(McIlveen[72])

There is no *larger, higher* quality RCT, with sufficient statistical analysis to support or refute the use of hydrotherapy rather than:
- other physiotherapy interventions
- other exercises.

Nominal group consensus

Hydrotherapy exercises may be more effective than no active intervention in:
- reducing pain (consensus 83%, second round) **IV**
- improving psychological status (consensus 83%, second round) **IV.**

Recommendations: hydrotherapy

Hydrotherapy exercises should be considered when aiming to:
- improve function   A
- reduce pain   C
- improve psychological status.   C

4.9   McKenzie exercises

Including exercise interventions organised according to McKenzie theory (see section 4.2 for definition of McKenzie exercises).

4.9.1 McKenzie exercises versus non-physiotherapy interventions

No RCTs comparing McKenzie exercises to non-physiotherapy interventions were found.

4.9.2 McKenzie exercises versus other physiotherapy interventions

No RCTs comparing McKenzie exercises to other physiotherapy interventions were found.

4.9.3 McKenzie exercises versus other exercises

One RCT was found: Petersen 2002[48].

Petersen's[48] *larger* (n=260) and *higher* methodological quality (6/10) trial found that a McKenzie programme compared with an intensive strengthening programme was:

- more effective in improving function (short-term) (but no difference immediately after intervention)

- similarly effective in improving function (long-term)

- similarly effective in reducing pain (short- and long-term)

- similarly effective in enabling return to work (short- and long-term).

Strengthening exercises reduce pain (section 4.4) and the effect of McKenzie exercises is similar, hence McKenzie exercises must also reduce pain. In the absence of research evidence that strengthening exercises improve function it is not possible to assume from Petersen's[48] trial (that compares McKenzie exercises with an unproven intervention) that McKenzie exercises improve function.

Evidence summary 7: McKenzie exercises

Research evidence

McKenzie therapy compared with a strengthening programme is:
- more effective in improving function (short-term), but no difference immediately after intervention **Ib**
- similarly effective in improving function (long-term) **Ib**
- similarly effective in reducing pain (short- and long-term) **Ib**
- similarly effective in enabling return to work (short- and long-term) **Ib**.

(Petersen[48])

There is no *larger, higher* quality RCT, with sufficient statistical analysis to support or refute the use of McKenzie exercises rather than:
- non-physiotherapy interventions
- other physiotherapy interventions.

Nominal group consensus

McKenzie exercises may be more effective than no active intervention in:
- improving function (consensus 87%, second round) **IV**
- improving psychological status (consensus 83%, second round) **IV**.

Recommendations: McKenzie exercises

McKenzie exercises should be considered when aiming to:
- reduce pain   A
- improve function   C
- improve psychological status.   C

4.10 Coordination exercises

One RCT was found: Johannsen 1995[57].

Johannsen's[57] trial (n=40) had a methodological quality of 1/10. The high attrition rate led to there being less than 15 participants per group for the final analysis.

Research evidence summary 8

Coordination exercises

There is no *larger, higher* quality RCT, with sufficient statistical analysis to support or refute the use of coordination exercises for persistent LBP.

Johansen's[57] trial is included here for completeness but in the GDG's experience coordination exercises are not a major component of physiotherapy interventions for people with persistent LBP. In the absence of evidence suggesting that this is a serious omission, coordination exercises are not referred to in the consensus questionnaire, which focuses on the major types of exercises used by physiotherapists.

4.11   Return to work

Three RCTs included in this review reported on return to work: Petersen 2002,[48] Hemmila 1997 and 2002[13, 14] and Joussett 2004[66].

Petersen's[48] trial was *larger* (n=260), of *higher* methodological quality (6/10) and found an intensive strengthening exercise programme, compared with a McKenzie therapy group, was:
- similarly effective in enabling return to work (short- and long-term).

Hemilla's[13, 14] trial (n=132) of *higher* methodological quality (7/10) found a general home exercise programme (strengthening and mobilising), compared with bone setting by traditional folk healers, was:
- similarly effective in reducing sick leave (short- and long-term).

Joussett's[66] trial (n=83) of methodological quality 4/10 compared an active individual therapy programme with a functional restoration programme. The results were inconclusive due to insufficient statistical analysis (section 2.6.4).

Research evidence summary 9

Research evidence

Intensive strengthening exercises compared with McKenzie therapy are:
- similarly effective in enabling return to work (short- and long-term) **Ib.**

Nominal group consensus

Not sought on this question; the GDG considered that the nominal group were not able to address this issue.

Thus there was an indication that both intensive strengthening and McKenzie therapy enabled return to work but the clinical question:

> Is exercise more effective in enabling return to work for people with persistent LBP than no active intervention?

could not be answered. The GDG looked to the European Guidelines for management of chronic LBP[6] for further evidence on this issue. Those guidelines concluded that:

> There is strong evidence that exercise therapy is more effective than 'general practitioner care' for ..... return to work in at least the mid-term (3-6 months). (p.84).

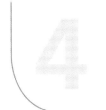

The European Guidelines found their evidence in the following trials: Lindstrom 1994,[73] 1992[74] and 1992[75] and, White 1969[76]. The Lindstrom paper was not included in this review because it considered a combination of interventions (section 2.6.2). The White paper was excluded because it considered people with specific diagnoses e.g., spondylolysis and herniated discs.

Recommendations: return to work

Evidence from a systematic review outside the scope of these guidelines suggests that exercise should be used to enable return to work   **not graded**

4.12   Cost effectiveness

Four RCTs have included a cost effectiveness analysis. Two were from the UK: Klaber Moffett 1999[58] and UK BEAM 2004[63, 64]. Two were from overseas Torstensen 1998[55] and Mannion 1999[56].

Klaber Moffett's[58] trial was *larger* (n=187) and of *higher* methodological quality (7/10). The mean total health care cost (i.e., all health care costs over 12 months including hospital visits and investigations etc.) per person, in 1999, for:

* the general exercise group was £360.15

* the standard general practitioner care group was £508.43.

The mean total cost (i.e., the intervention specific care for back pain over 12 months) per person, in 1999, was, for:

* the general exercise group, £86.83

* the standard general practitioner care group, £111.05.

The UK BEAM trial[63, 64] was *larger* (n=1334) and of *higher* methodological quality (6/10). It reported that the mean total costs for all health care patients in each group was:

* exercise with general practitioner care £486 per year

* manipulation with general practitioner care £541 per year

* general practitioner care alone £346 per year.

In this trial health care costs for back pain were not separated from other health care costs.

Torstensen's[55] *larger* (n=208) and *higher* methodological quality trial (8/10) included a cost analysis and was conducted in Norway. The direct costs of sick leave (over a 15 month period) were the lowest for the physical mixed methods group (5,980,200 Norwegian kroner (NOK)), followed by the general exercises group (7,054,200 NOK) and highest for the walking programme (8,152,200 NOK). However the direct costs of the treatment were lowest for the walking group (0 NOK), followed by the general exercises group (2772 NOK) and highest for the physical mixed methods group (4320 NOK).

Mannion's[56] *larger* (n=148) and *higher* methodological quality trial (9/10) was conducted in Switzerland and reported mean health care costs per person. The group that followed a general aerobic exercise programme had the lowest costs (288 SFr), the physical mixed methods group had higher mean costs (960 SFr) but the exercise group, which used various sophisticated devices (David Black exercise equipment), was the most expensive (1120 SFr).

The nominal consensus group discussed the cost of group exercise (appendix E2). There was GDG consensus that group exercise reduces the cost per person. At the same time, where people with persistent LBP are comfortable with this approach, they gain peer support and thus improved confidence and empowerment to manage with less medical intervention.

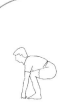

Research evidence summary 10

Cost effectiveness of exercise

- Overall costs during a 12 month period were less for a general exercise programme ('back to fitness') compared with general practitioner care only. The outcome in terms of pain reduction and improved function was better for the exercise group **Ib**

- Exercise is more expensive than general practitioner care alone, in terms of total health care costs over 12 months. The outcome in terms of pain reduction, improved function and decreased fear avoidance is better for the group that included exercise **Ib**

- Unsupervised walking is a low cost exercise option. The outcome in terms of reduced pain and improved function is worse than for a supervised general exercise group **Ib**

- Exercises that involve sophisticated equipment are more expensive. The outcome is similar to exercising without expensive equipment **Ib.**

GDG consensus

- Group exercise reduces the cost per person. The outcome is likely to be better in terms of peer support thus giving people improved confidence and empowering them to manage with less medical intervention **IV.**

Recommendations: cost effectiveness

- Exercise is recommended to reduce pain and improve function   A
- The use of sophisticated equipment is not necessary   A
- Unsupervised walking is low in cost   A
- Where feasible, and acceptable in terms of patient choice, group exercise is recommended to reduce costs e.g., group hydrotherapy may be cost effective.   D

4.13 Safety

The included RCTs did not report any safety issues relating to exercise interventions for persistent low back pain.

Research evidence summary 11

Safety of exercise interventions

There is no *larger, higher* quality RCT, with sufficient statistical analysis to support or refute the safety of exercises as an intervention for people with persistent LBP.

Recommendations: safety

- Physiotherapists should be aware of all the health and safety issues relevant to their patient population and their work place.   D

4.14   Exercise in combination with another intervention

Readers should note that RCTs considering the effectiveness of exercise **in combination** with another physiotherapy intervention (e.g., exercise and electrotherapy or exercise and massage) are excluded from this review. These studies cannot assist in answering the major clinical question (section 1.2). The process by which knowledge about the effectiveness of a single intervention can be extracted from a complex study of this nature is beyond the scope of these guidelines. Some studies, familiar to the GDG, that fall into this classification are:

- Deyo (1990)[77]
- Frost (1998)[78]
- Klein (1990)[79]
- Lidstrom and Zachrisson (1970).[80]

Further details of all excluded trials are given in the appendices (appendix D, table 4).

A pragmatic decision was taken where exercises are combined with a second non-physiotherapy intervention e.g., the UK BEAM trial[63, 64] (compared exercise in combination with general practitioner care). The majority of people with persistent LBP attending physiotherapy clinics are likely to have consulted a general practitioner hence this trial was included.

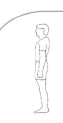

4.15   Evidence summaries

Reducing pain for people with persistent LBP

Type of exercise	Type of evidence	Grade of evidence	Found in
Mobilising exercises	Insufficient research evidence to support or refute	No evidence	Evidence summary 1
	Effective (consensus 83%, second round)	IV	
Strengthening exercises	Effective (research evidence)	Ib	Evidence summary 2
Unsupervised walking	Insufficient research evidence to support or refute	No evidence	Evidence summary 3
	Insufficient consensus evidence to support or refute		
Organised aerobic exercises	Effective (research evidence)	Ib	
General exercises	Effective (research evidence)	Ib	Evidence summary 4
Core stability exercises	Insufficient research evidence to support or refute	No evidence	Evidence summary 5
	Insufficient consensus evidence to support or refute		
Hydrotherapy exercises	Insufficient research evidence to support or refute	No evidence	Evidence summary 6
	Effective (consensus 83%, second round)	IV	
McKenzie exercises	Effective (research evidence)	Ib	Evidence summary 7

Improving function for people with persistent LBP

Type of exercise	Type of evidence	Grade of evidence	Found in
Mobilising exercises	Not identified in this literature search	No evidence	Evidence summary 1
	Effective (consensus 91%, second round)	IV	
Strengthening exercises	Insufficient research evidence to support or refute	No evidence	Evidence summary 2
	Effective (consensus 80%, first round)	IV	
Unsupervised walking	Insufficient research evidence to support or refute	No evidence	Evidence summary 3
	Effective (consensus 76%, first round)	IV	
Organised aerobic exercises	Effective (research evidence)	Ib	
General exercises	Effective (research evidence)	Ib	Evidence summary 4
Core stability exercises	Insufficient research evidence to support or refute	No evidence	Evidence summary 5
	Effective (consensus 83%, second round)	IV	
Hydrotherapy exercises	Effective (research evidence)	Ib	Evidence summary 6
McKenzie exercises	Insufficient research evidence to support or refute	No evidence	Evidence summary 7
	Effective (consensus 87%, second round)	IV	

Improving psychological status for people with persistent LBP

Type of exercise	Type of evidence	Grade of evidence	Found in
Mobilising exercises	Not identified in this literature search	No evidence	Evidence summary 1
	Effective (consensus 83%, second round)	IV	
Strengthening exercises	Not identified in this literature search	No evidence	Evidence summary 2
	Effective (consensus 87%, second round)	IV	
Unsupervised walking	Not identified in this literature search	No evidence	Evidence summary 3
	Effective (consensus 84%, first round)	IV	
Organised aerobic exercises	Insufficient research evidence to support or refute	No evidence	
	Effective (consensus 96%, first round)	IV	
General exercises	Insufficient research evidence to support or refute	No evidence	Evidence summary 4
	Effective (consensus 88%, first round)	IV	
Core stability exercises	Insufficient research evidence to support or refute	No evidence	Evidence summary 5
	Insufficient consensus evidence to support or refute		
Hydrotherapy exercises	Not identified in this literature search	No evidence	Evidence summary 6
	Effective (consensus 83%, second round)	IV	
McKenzie exercises	Not identified in this literature search	No evidence	Evidence summary 7
	Effective (consensus 83%, second round)	IV	

There is research evidence that hydrotherapy exercises improve function for people with persistent LBP but this question also went to consensus because the research evidence had not been found at the time of sending out the consensus questionnaire. The research evidence is of a *higher* level and hence takes priority over the consensus evidence.

Return to work for people with persistent LBP

Type of exercise	Type of evidence	Grade of evidence	Found in
Unspecific	An indication that strengthening exercises and McKenzie exercises may both be effective	No evidence	Evidence summary 9
	Consensus was not sought on this issue because it was felt to be outside the GDG's expertise		
	Strong evidence from the European guidelines that exercise is effective but including groups of people not considered here	Not graded	

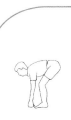

Cost effectiveness

Type of exercise	Type of evidence	Grade of evidence	Found in
General exercise	Effective (research evidence)	Ib	Evidence summary 10

Safety

Type of exercise	Type of evidence	Grade of evidence	Found in
Unspecific	Not addressed in the literature	**No evidence**	Evidence summary 11
	Consensus was not sought on this issue because it was felt to be outside the GDG's expertise		

5 The clinical recommendations

These recommendations are derived from the systematic review (grade **A**), the results of the nominal group consensus questionnaire (grade **C**) and GDG consensus (grade **D**). The grade **D** recommendations are derived from discussion (e.g., the consensus conference appendix E2 and GDG meetings) and they assist in applying the grade **A** and **C** recommendation to various clinical settings.

It should be emphasised that no evidence was sought to demonstrate the superiority of one type of exercise over another; there was no evidence of its existence. At the same time, there is no grade **B** evidence because the GDG made a pragmatic decision to include RCTs only in the systematic review.

To emphasise the source of the evidence for each recommendation the summary table from section 2.9 is reproduced (table 2.4).

Table 2.4 Grading guideline recommendations adapted from NICE[16]

Grade	Evidence
A	At least one RCT of overall higher quality and consistency addressing the specific recommendation (evidence levels Ia and Ib in Table 2.1)
B	Well-conducted clinical studies but not RCTs on the topic of the recommendation (evidence levels IIa, IIb and III in Table 2.1)
C	Evidence from the nominal group technique or other expert committee reports. This indicates that directly applicable clinical studies or higher quality are absent (evidence level IV in Table 2.1)
D	Recommended good practice based on the clinical experience of the GDG

5.1 Supervised exercises

The key clinical recommendation is:

People with persistent LBP should be given the opportunity to participate in an exercise programme, in a form appropriate and acceptable to each individual, after physiotherapy assessment — A

To **reduce pain** one or more of the following should be considered:
- Strengthening exercises — A
- Organised aerobic exercises — A
- General exercises — A
- McKenzie exercises — A
- Mobilising exercises — C
- Hydrotherapy exercises — C

To **improve function** one or more of the following should be considered:
- Organised aerobic exercises — A
- General exercises — A
- Hydrotherapy exercises — A
- Mobilising exercises — C
- Strengthening exercises — C

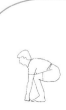

- Core stability exercises   C
- McKenzie exercises   C

To **improve psychological** status one or more of the following should be considered:
- Mobilising exercises   C
- Strengthening exercises   C
- Organised aerobic exercises   C
- General exercises   C
- Hydrotherapy exercises   C
- McKenzie exercises   C

5.2   Application of supervised exercises

The above recommendations are general points that reflect the research evidence and the consensus evidence. Exercise is beneficial. However people are individuals and GDG discussion led to the following recommendations.

5.2.1   The individual

- **Individual assessment** is essential before embarking on any physiotherapy   D
  intervention and this includes exercise programmes (section 3)

- **Individual health status** should be considered when choosing the type and pace of   D
  an exercise intervention e.g., a person with osteoporosis would need a different
  programme to a competitive athlete with high bone density

- **Individual lifestyle** should be considered when choosing an exercise intervention e.g.,   D
  the goal may be return to work but an office worker will need a different programme
  to a person with a heavy manual job

- **Psychosocial assessment** of people's beliefs and willingness to participate in a   D
  particular exercise programme should be carried out before referral to that programme

- **Grading and pacing of exercises** to a suitable level for the individual is essential e.g.,   D
  unsuitable high intensity exercise may result in increased pain and fear avoidance

- **Patient choice** should affect choice of exercises e.g., believing in the benefits of   D
  aerobic exercises should suggest aerobic exercises as a first choice of exercise programme

- **Patient involvement** in actively managing their persistent LBP should be encouraged   D
  where appropriate e.g., a person interested in joining a local general exercise group
  should be encouraged with this

- **Patient expectations** should always be considered in choice of exercise to maximise   D
  outcome e.g., a person who expects supervised exercise should be encouraged to join a
  suitable exercise class rather than encouraged to walk or swim independently.

5.2.2 Resources

- **Resources at the place of treatment** will affect choice of exercises e.g., hydrotherapy exercises can only be given where a person can access pool facilities   D

- **Resources at the person's home** should affect choice of exercises e.g., expensive equipment should not be relied upon where a person is advised to continue with their programme at home if they do not have suitable equipment at home   D

- **Resources in the person's community** should affect choice of exercises e.g., a local swimming pool with a self-help hydrotherapy group may suggest hydrotherapy exercises as a first choice of treatment   D

- **Local human resources** should affect choice of exercises e.g., a local community centre might have an expert in aerobic exercise suggesting that aerobic exercises may be a first choice of treatment.   D

5.2.3 The practitioner

- **The special interest or training of the practitioner** affects the choice of exercises and this should be made explicit to people with persistent LBP e.g., a physiotherapist with additional McKenzie training is more likely than colleagues without specialist training to recommend this exercise intervention   D

- **The confidence and experience of the practitioner** is important e.g., experts teaching exercises with conviction are likely to achieve the best outcomes and this should be recognised.   D

5.2.4 Advice

- **Advice and education** given by the practitioner should be appropriate and evidence based. Some main points drawn from sources outside the scope of these guidelines are: not graded (section 5.6)
    - movement is beneficial for your back
    - there is unlikely to be any serious damage to your back
    - your pain is likely to improve in the short-term although it is likely to recur
    - simple painkillers are likely to help reduce the pain
    - your back is strong
    - staying at work / continuing with usual activity is normally helpful

    (Section 7 gives more detail of advice).

- Unsupervised walking

    People may be advised of the benefits of unsupervised walking in:
    - improving function   C
    - imroving psychological status   C

Psychosocial factors may adversely affect involvement, and where unsupervised walking is recommended it should always be with suitable advise on pacing.   D

5.3 Return to work

- Evidence from a systematic review outside the scope of these guidelines suggests that exercise should be used to enable return to work.

  not graded
  (section 5.6)

5.4 Cost effectiveness

- Exercise is recommended to reduce pain and improve function   A
- The use of sophisticated equipment is not necessary   A
- Unsupervised walking is low in cost   A
- Where feasible, and acceptable in terms of patient choice, group exercise is recommended to reduce costs e.g., group hydrotherapy may be cost effective.   D

5.5 Safety

- Physiotherapists should be aware of all health and safety issues relevant to their patient population and their work place.   D

5.6 Further points to note

- Where recommendations rely on evidence outside the scope of our systematic review, nominal group consensus exercise or GDG expertise they are not graded

- No recommendations are made about core stability exercises and either pain reduction or improvement in psychological status. This is because no evidence was found in these areas. However the GDG are aware of recent research in this area

- No recommendations are made about unsupervised walking and pain reduction. Again no evidence was found in this area but GDG consensus stresses the benefit of this activity in improving both function and psychological status

- The GDG suggest further literature that may assist researchers interested in section 5.2.3 considering the practitioner.[81-85]

6 Research recommendations

The evidence from both research and expert opinion is unequivocal; exercise is beneficial for people with persistent LBP. Nevertheless there are gaps in the research evidence and attention should be given to addressing these. At the same time, the GDG recommend that physiotherapists consider wider research questions as outlined below. Furthermore these guidelines have highlighted methodological insufficiencies with many RCTs and the GDG recommend that attention be given to ensuring rigorous methodology in future trials.

6.2 Research questions

Where possible the questions below include a population, intervention, comparison and an outcome (PICO) as recommended by the National Institute of Clinical Excellence (NICE) (http://www.nice.org.uk/page.aspx?o=247851). For some questions 'general practitioner care' has been used as a comparison but any non-active intervention e.g., a waiting list control might be substituted.

6.2.1 Questions relating to the sub-classification of people with LBP

Much current research focuses on sub-classification of people with LBP and the GDG suggests that this is an important area of work. The variation in causes of LBP may explain why many *smaller* trials fail to either show statistically or clinically significant results. Future comparisons might go beyond age, gender, duration of complaints, severity of complaints, and sick leave as studied to date, to explore different levels of psychological distress or different patient expectations. The GDG suggest that the key research question is:

Are there identifiable sub-groups of people with persistent LBP who respond best to particular types of exercise?

Recommendations for questions in this area are:

Does the **level of psychological distress** affect the outcome (in terms of pain, function, psychological status and return to work) of a general exercise programme, for people with persistent LBP?

Do **patient expectations** affect the outcome (in terms of pain, function, psychological status and return to work) of a general exercise programme, for people with persistent LBP?

Can we **predict the outcome** for any particular subgroup of people e.g., according to psychological distress, patient expectations, presence of leg pain?

In addition to RCTs, because this work is in an initial stage (section 6.3), studies using alternative methods are required, for example:
• Reliability studies to identify reproducible methods of assessment or classification
• Cohort studies to identify sub-groups that have prognostic validity
• Sub-group trials to identify the most effective intervention.

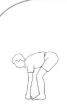

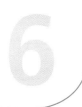

6.2.2 Other priority research questions

The evidence is that exercise is effective but there are some aspects of supervised exercise that require further investigation.

Does participation in an exercise programme, compared with general practitioner care, speed **return to work** for people with persistent LBP?

Does participation in an exercise programme, compared with general practitioner care, improve **psychological status** for people with persistent LBP?

At the same time there are other important gaps in the literature that need addressing.

- Is it necessary to focus interventions directly to treating **psychological status** to improve psychological status?
- Are **specific exercises**, compared with non-specific exercises, more effective in improving pain, function, psychological status and return to work for people with persistent LBP?
- Does **unsupervised exercise** (e.g., walking, cycling, swimming) compared with general practitioner care, improve pain, function, psychological status and return to work for people with persistent LBP?
- Does **group exercise** or **individual exercise** lead to greater improvement in pain, function, psychological status and return to work for people with persistent LBP?
- How do physiotherapists perceive the effect of **patient choice** on the outcome of exercise?
- **How does exercise work?** E.g., to what extent do strengthening exercises, for people with persistent LBP, increase muscle strength, and to what extent do they increase well being and confidence?
- Have these guidelines been successfully **implemented** into clinical practice and what effect have they had on practice?

6.3 Methodological considerations

There are two phases (see paragraphs below) in the process of evaluating the effectiveness of an intervention, they are different in approach but both are essential. Once the second phase is reached the first phase must continue as interventions develop and the knowledge base grows.

The first phase may be during development of a new intervention. At this stage a small group of participants is often sufficient and results are used to refine the intervention and/or to develop the science behind it. An initial exploratory stage is always essential. All physiotherapists can be involved in research in this phase, examples of activity are:
- single case studies as a continuing professional development (CPD) activity
- audit of a single service to assess outcome
- small qualitative studies asking specific questions
- pilot studies as a precursor to large multicentre randomised trials.

A research active profession is critical both for the implementation of current evidence and to ensure the future evidence base of physiotherapy.

In the second phase demonstrating that the intervention works becomes the important aim. Initial results are reproduced in *larger*, probably multi-centred studies using rigorous research methods. Unlike the initial studies the results of these studies can form a solid basis for recommendations for practice. In theory it is possible to collate the results of a series of *smaller* studies to form a solid base for recommendations but in practice variation in interventions, participants and methods make this a less robust approach.

The GDG recommend that RCTs should always be of the highest possible quality. Those considering setting up RCTs should always ensure that they:

- are of the highest possible methodological quality

- give detail to enable the reader to understand the interventions or procedures used

- use relevant outcome measures (section 3.7, section 4 and the measures recommended for clinical trials of chronic pain[29])

- include a sufficient number of participants; a sample size calculation is essential; multi-centre trials are more likely to be in a position to recruit more participants and have the further advantage of increased external validity (generalisability)

- include appropriate statistical analysis to identify any differences in effectiveness between intervention groups.

In addition, quality reporting of studies is of paramount importance. It is the paper that is scored and not the process thus poor reporting leads to low scores. Details about conducting quality RCTs are available from the CONSORT **website: http://www.consort-statement.org/**

A final consideration is that 'standard physiotherapy' may not be a suitable intervention for a RCT comparison group. The GDG found it extremely difficult to interpret trials using this comparison group when assessing the outcomes of physiotherapy intervention. A major problem was that minimal information was given about the interventions received by the 'standard physiotherapy' group making conclusions vague and unspecific.

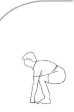

7 Advice and education for people with persistent LBP

Health professionals and educational material should always give consistent messages[7] Although advice and education are outside the scope of this systematic review some material from other sources is cited because advice and education are vital to every therapist-patient interaction. The sources, which give further information, are:

- The Back Pain Revolution[7]
- The Back Book[52]
- Working backs Scotland: www.workingbacksscotland.com
- BackCare: http://www.backcare.org.uk/
- A People's Guide to Active Backcare.[86]

As with assessment (section 3) readers are again recommended to access the information sources given above. This section outlines the basic messages for people with persistent LBP. The messages given here represent both current thinking and GDG consensus.

7.1 The nature of the pain

- It is likely to improve
- It is likely to recur. Attacks may settle over several years but the pain may be ongoing (chronic pain). One third of people with chronic back pain improve spontaneously
- The greatest risk factor for back pain is previous history of back pain as its natural history is to recur.
- Movement may cause pain but this should not be seen as damage and should not be avoided
- Back pain is almost universal and most people will get back pain at some time
- Being tall, fat, thin or having unequal leg length does not inevitably lead to back pain
- Back pain will not inevitably lead to chronic pain and disability
- Being generally healthy e.g., giving up smoking, avoiding excessive weight and being physically fit will not mean that people avoid back pain but it will help them to deal with it better.

7.2 Living with the pain

- Movement is good for the back and is likely to help the pain
- Regular simple painkillers can help manage pain (advice should be sought from a doctor or pharmacist or follow instructions on the packet)
- A cold pack or hot pack might be useful to help relieve pain in the short-term.
- Do not sit or stand in one position for too long; change position often
- Get up and walk about to avoid stiffening up
- Take regular breaks e.g., when driving or sitting
- Always remember that the structures in the back are strong.

7.3 Work and normal activity

- It is important to stay active and continue as normally as possible. It may hurt and cause discomfort but aim to get back to normal as quickly as possible

- Movement will help speed recovery

- Keeping the back moving stops it from stiffening up. Working through initial discomfort will speed returning to normal

- Try to stay at work, or return to work quickly even if there is still some pain. Getting back to work (or normal activity) can help faster recovery. Staying off work (or normal activity) longer increases likelihood of developing chronic pain and disability

- Many people find they can continue most activities despite the pain but some things may take a little longer or need to be done a different way

- Some things may be more difficult with back pain, but back pain is not usually caused by work.

- Walking and swimming are good forms of regular exercise

- Usually, people will find that work is beneficial for pain. It is unlikely to be helpful to stay off work, change jobs or give up work completely, because of ordinary back pain. Manual work does not necessarily cause back injury or degenerative changes, although it might aggravate back pain

- Aim to be as comfortable and safe as possible at work by preventing excessive fatigue, discomfort and stress.

What causes ongoing back pain?

The causes of back pain are not yet clearly understood, and may involve many factors. Nevertheless it is possible to make some suggestions.

- Physical factors (biomechanical) (e.g., manual handling, lifting, bending twisting, repetitive movements, static work postures, sitting, driving) might contribute to back pain. But psychosocial issues probably affect the impact and consequences

- When people have their first episode of back pain it is probably not possible to tell who may develop chronic pain. The critical period is 4-12 weeks post-onset; at this stage the psychosocial factors can become more important in the development of chronic disability. At this stage we should try to identify those at risk and intervene. By 12 weeks post-onset people still off work are at high risk of long-term incapacity. At this stage the obstacles to recovery and return to work urgently need addressing.

7.4 General strategy of advice

- *Reassure* that there is no serious damage or disease

- *Explain* back pain as a part of human experience

- *Avoid* labelling the pain as injury, disc trouble, wear and tear or any label that might imply that rest rather than activity is helpful

- *Reassure* about good natural history, providing you stay active, but give accurate information about recurrent symptoms and how to deal with them

- *Advise* on the use of simple, safe treatments to control symptoms (e.g., simple painkillers – follow instructions, a cold pack or local heat)

- *Encourage* staying active, continuing daily activities as normally as possible, and staying at work. This gives the most rapid and complete recovery and less risk of recurrent problems

- *Avoid* 'let pain be your guide' without instruction on pacing

- *Encourage* people to take responsibility for their own continued management.[7]

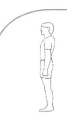

8 Implementation

8.1 Background

Implementation of clinical guidelines involves their planned and systematic introduction into clinical practice[87]. It is clinicians and their patients who implement recommendations although policy-makers, managers, professional bodies, educators and managers can promote the use of guidelines.

8.2 Potential barriers and facilitators

Implementation is complex because there are many barriers to change and these are discussed below with an indication of how the CSP, clinicians and patients, and managers can assist in the process.

8.2.1 Knowledge barriers

Knowledge of the existence of guidelines and thus the recommendations made may be limited[88].

The CSP will promote an awareness of the availability of these guidelines to all members through, for example:
- articles in 'Frontline' and other relevant publications
- the interactive CSP (iCSP) website
- promoting the guideline at CSP congress and other relevant conferences
- liasing with relevant clinical interest and occupational groups.

8.2.2 Organisational barriers (including time)

Time limitations, difficulties in communication and collaboration with other healthcare practitioners have been identified as barriers to the use of guidelines in physiotherapy.[87, 88] Clinicians need time to appraise guidelines, to discuss the recommendations and consider the implications for implementation.

Managers are encouraged to support clinicians in activities such as:
- discussion groups to break down barriers across different practice settings (including private practice)
- educational support activities with protected time.

8.2.3 Cost and access

Studies have shown that physiotherapists have difficulty in obtaining copies of guidelines or they share one copy amongst many colleagues which may be frustrating.[88]

The CSP plan to continue their policy of keeping the cost of guidelines low for members. The CSP will also produce a quick reference guide to summarise the recommendations and thus will assist practitioners working with patients.

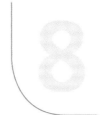

8.2.4   Practitioner factors

These include the beliefs and attitudes of clinicians, the skills of individual clinicians, the influence of opinion leaders[89] and the local experience of adapting practice to national guidelines. A frequently reported barrier to implementation of guidelines relates to a lack of knowledge or skills in the target group of clinicians[87, 88].

Managers and clinicians are encouraged to address these barriers through:
- continuing professional development and education
- recognising the link between implementing these guidelines and evidence based practice.

8.2.5   Patient expectations

It is becoming increasingly clear that patients' beliefs and expectations of treatment influence outcome.[90-92] Patients' expectations may act as a barrier to guideline implementation as many patients have preferences for interventions now considered outdated or ineffective.

Clinicians are encouraged to recognise the importance of involving patients in clinical decision making when using clinical guidelines in practice.[93] For example clinicians may discuss, with individuals, the recommendations for practice and how they might apply personally.

8.3   Research and implementation

Research is needed to:
- study the effectiveness of guideline implementation strategies, particularly in health professions other than medicine (e.g., Evans 2005[94]).
- demonstrate that implementing guideline recommendations improves patient outcomes (e.g., Feuerstein 2006[95]).

8.4   Implementing these guidelines

It should be emphasised that nationally developed guidelines will necessarily undergo a level of local adaptation at the implementation stage.

These guidelines contribute to the management of people with persistent LBP as they:
- give a level of detail about exercise for persistent LBP not available elsewhere
- critically appraise the literature to emphasise the research findings from *larger, higher* quality research studies with robust statistical analysis
- give recommendations by an expert team where the research evidence is lacking in a way that has not been attempted in other guidelines.

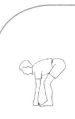

8

To assist in implementing these guidelines the following additional documents have been produced:

- **A quick reference guide**. It is intended that practitioners carry these in their workplace as a reminder of the recommendations for practice (see fold-out in back cover)
- **An audit pack** (see insert in front cover). This is to assist practitioners in comparing actual practice with the recommendations in the guidelines.

Advice on conducting the audit can be found elsewhere e.g., CSP's Osteoporosis Audit Pack (2002)[96] and the NICE Principles of Best Practice in Clinical Audit (2002).[97]

9   Updating these guidelines

9.1   The planned update

It is planned that these guidelines will be updated in 2011.

At the time of publishing, the CSP's process for producing and updating guidelines is under review and therefore this date may change and/or the format of future documents may be different.

9.2   Review of the guideline development programme

In early 2006, after seven years of running the guidelines programme, this review aimed to clarify what had been learned, understand CSP member's perceptions of the programme, and inform future working. The review found that the work in the guidelines programme was valued and overwhelmingly supported. Nevertheless there were process problems and these were addressed in the review's recommendations.

This review recommended that the CSP should:
- develop a framework of clear processes to enable the production of information to support physiotherapy practice
- establish an online database for this clinical practice information
- engage CSP members in developing the information that they need for their practice
- use the framework for developing all evidence based clinical practice information e.g., systematic reviews, evidence briefings and guidelines
- devise an implementation programme for clinical practice information that seeks to empower clinicians and managers.

Further information about the review can be found on the effective practice network of iCSP:
www.interactivecsp.org.uk

9.3   Supporting knowledge in physiotherapy practice project (SKIPP)

The CSP has accepted the above recommendations and, at the time of writing, the research and clinical effectiveness unit has set up a project team to take this work forwards.

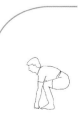

10

10 GDG reflection

10.1 The evidence base

The GDG acknowledges the paucity of strong evidence in terms of many types of exercise intervention for people with persistent LBP and their consequent reliance on expert clinical experience in developing these guidelines. As more research is carried out, the recommendations will be modified and become more robust. Nevertheless, at the time of writing, the best available evidence is presented, and interpreted, in the light of current knowledge. Further the GDG has drawn on research evidence from different fields including psychology and sports sciences.

10.2 Some difficult decisions

In producing these guidelines the GDG had to make some difficult decisions and some examples are given here. In the early stages it was unclear how 'persistent' LBP should be defined. When writing the scope 'persistent' was defined as three months or more (appendix A). However it soon became apparent that rigidly applying this definition would exclude a great deal of the literature that included participants with a shorter duration of LBP. Hence a pragmatic decision was made to redefine 'persistent' as six weeks or more.

At a later stage, it was decided that it was clinically relevant to consider the different types of exercise used by physiotherapists but it was difficult to decide on how to categorise some of the trials. For example, Koumantakis's trial[49] was originally included in the general exercise section but was finally included in both the strengthening exercises section (4.4.3) and in the core stability exercises section (4.7.3).

A further difficult decision was whether the UK BEAM trial[63, 64] (relevant, *larger* and *higher* in methodological quality) could be included in the evidence review because a decision had been made to exclude trials that considered exercise in combination with another intervention from this evidence review (section 4.14). After much debate it was decided to include this trial, which considered exercise in combination with general practitioner care, because the majority of people with persistent LBP attending physiotherapy are also consulting a general practitioner.

10.3 Focusing on the evidence review

This section considers decisions made during the process of the evidence review i.e., the literature, the assessment of methodological quality, data extraction, assessment of sample size and outcomes measures.

10.3.1 The literature

There is much literature relating to LBP and this led to a pragmatic decision to limit the literature search to RCTs, which provide the most reliable study design to test effectiveness of an intervention. Where there were no RCTs fulfilling our criteria on methodological quality, statistical rigour and sample size (section 2.6) then statements derived from the nominal group technique were used to make recommendations. The nominal group was asked to base their decision on their knowledge of the literature (including non-RCT evidence) and their experience. Non-RCT evidence was not used in the

evidence review because the budget and resources available for this project did not allow examination of the estimated 5000 articles identified in the initial literature search.

10.3.2 Assessment of methodological quality

Any scale necessarily gives a simplification of the true methodological quality of a RCT. The GDG chose 10 items from the original 24 items of the van Tulder Quality Scale[10] in order to assess the internal validity of the RCTs. In addition the GDG assessed:

- statistical quality by including only RCTs that presented statistics directly comparing change in the intervention group with change in a comparison group (section 2.6.4)

- sample size by including those with 40 or more participants in the intervention group (section 2.6.5)

- descriptive quality by several methods: the inclusion criteria (section 2.6.2), description of interventions, description of adverse effects (appendix D, tables 1 and 3).

One change was made to the 10 criteria of the adapted van Tulder Quality Scale used by the GDG; an item comparing the groups at baseline replaced an item concerning outcome measures. The GDG considered that relevance of outcomes was dealt with by the structure of the evidence tables (i.e., only outcomes on pain, function, psychological status and return to work/ sick leave were included (appendix D, tables 3a-e). At the same time, similarity of baseline values was not assessed elsewhere.

Two independent reviewers assessed methodological quality. Disagreements on the scores were solved by discussion. No statistics are available for the level of agreement between the two reviewers but it is suggested that this analysis might be included in future reviews.

10.3.3 Data extraction

The data extraction was conducted by two reviewers who resolved differences through discussion. A strict structure for data extraction was used (appendix D) and although this led to some data being disregarded it allowed the GDG to address the specific clinical questions (section 2.5).

10.3.4 Assessment of sample size

Ideally a power analysis is used to determine sample size but in most instances these were not included in the papers and could not be calculated by the GDG (section 2.6.5). Defining sample size as '*larger*' (or by implication '*smaller*') is a simplification but there is evidence that large samples sizes (up to n=60 per intervention group) are needed to obtain statistically significant changes in pain in drug trials.[12] These numbers are needed because chance affects variability in pain response. There is no evidence about the sample sizes needed in physiotherapy studies but it is likely that they would need to be of a similar size to those used in drug trials. For that reason a pragmatic approach was used and trials were defined as *larger* where there were 40 or more participants in the intervention group.

To justify this position, decreasing the definition of *larger* trials to 30 participants per intervention group would have resulted in redefining only two trials:

- Storheim et al (2003)[54]

- and Tritilanunt et al (2001).[43]

Both these RCTs considered the use of aerobic exercises for which level **Ib** evidence already existed (Mannion et al 1999[56]). Thus the recommendations of these guidelines would have been unchanged.

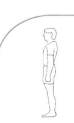

On the other hand, increasing the definition of *larger* trial to 50 participants per intervention group would have excluded many RCTs from this review and this seemed too rigid an approach for the evidence. The GDG recognise that future updates using new research evidence are likely to make different decisions.

10.3.5 Outcome measures

Further to all the discussion on trial quality and size, findings are only as valid and reliable as the outcome measures that they use. For this reason the GDG sought to assess the validity, reliability and relevance of the outcome measures used in the trials that led to the level **Ib** evidence (appendix H). The conclusion was that the outcome measures were appropriate, indeed many researchers used measures recommended by the GDG (section 3.7). This emphasises the robust evidence base for the recommendations made in these guidelines.

10.4   Focusing on the Methods

In July 2005 it was agreed that the original scope of these guidelines was impractically broad and that an initial publication would consider exercise alone. Following this the final draft of the exercise evidence review was completed in November 2005 and these guidelines went out to review in February 2006.

The GDG worked to streamline the guideline development process (section 2.1) while maintaining a high scientific standard. The advantages are twofold:
- guidelines are produced before the evidence review is out of date
- the costs of producing guidelines is reduced.

Below are some of the innovative methods used by this GDG and some further reflection on these methods.

10.4.1 Telephone conferences for GDG meetings

GDG meetings, held at approximately two monthly intervals from July 2005, were all telephone conferences. This had several advantages:
- time was saved and travel time was eliminated
- the costs of the meetings were greatly reduced
- meetings were extremely focussed and decisions reached quickly and where more discussion was needed this was by electronic means
- attendance at meetings was generally high
- more regular meetings were possible thus expediting guideline production.

10.4.2 Consensus questionnaires were sent out and returned by email

Both rounds of the consensus questionnaires were sent out and returned by email and on both occasions two weeks were allocated to the process. As a comparison, each round of the consensus questionnaires for the CSP guidelines for the management of whiplash associated disorder were sent out and returned by post and took between 4 and 6 weeks.[18]

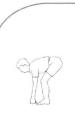

10.4.3 The consensus conference was held on the iCSP

The nominal group consensus conference took place electronically. Each question to be discussed was posted on the iCSP's 'discussion forum' and the nominal consensus group were given two weeks to make their points and read the views of their peers. Group members suggested the following advantages to this iCSP conference, they:

- had time to consider their response

- could join the conference when it suited them

- were able to see a record of people's comments.

On the other hand:

- some group members felt that it was difficult to keep track of different parts of the iCSP site but the new iCSP site, launched in March 2006, should be clearer.

In addition, using the record of the discussion, it was an easy step to add an outline of the discussion to the guidelines (appendix E2). This appendix is intended to increase the transparency of the consensus process and gives some background to the shift towards greater agreement in the nominal consensus group (appendix E4). Further the outline of the discussion indicates the origin of the GDG recommendations for good practice (section 5.2) that were reworded at the GDG meeting on 9th February 2006.

10.4.4 Some discussion was also by email

In association with the iCSP discussion email was used. For example, after the GDG meeting of 9th February 2006 when the topics for the research recommendations were suggested two drafts of this section (6.0) were discussed by email. In general the group felt that email gave them:

- another means for having discussion

- a quicker response because messages arrived directly into people's in-trays

- an alternative means of communication which was helpful.

To further increase transparency, a flavour of the email discussion that led to the research recommendations (section 6) has been added to this final document (appendix E5) to indicate how the group agreed these recommendations.

10.5   Selection of GDG members

The members of the GDG were carefully chosen to represent, as broadly as possible, physiotherapy expertise in LBP. The initial scoping exercise (appendix A) revealed the range of people to be represented (appendix B). These guidelines were developed over a lengthy period of time and this resulted in changes in GDG membership. New members were invited to join the group because they had similar skills to a retiring member; they were made aware of the scope of the guidelines and the framework in which they would work.

The aim was to develop physiotherapy specific guidelines and for this reason it was not a major issue that other professional groups were under represented. There was a sports scientist GDG member but budget constraints meant that we were unable to recruit a general practitioner, a psychologist or a private practitioner. Nevertheless it is acknowledged that the content of these guidelines are likely to be useful for non-physiotherapists involved in the treatment of LBP.

10.6   Patient representation

The GDG included one patient representative, Nia Taylor, Chief executive of BackCare. No further representation was sought as Nia's role and personal experience of back pain ensured effective representation. Nia Taylor's experience is outlined below:

- She has experienced back pain, once quite severely and then intermittently, and was referred to a physiotherapist by her general practitioner. She continues to use the exercises that her physiotherapist taught her if her back pain flares up. Thus she has experience in self managing her own back pain

- As chief executive of BackCare she is in regular contact with many people living with back pain. She discusses the issues that people with back pain raise with the BackCare helpline manager and the helpline volunteers. She personally answers telephone, written and email enquiries to BackCare

- She is chair of the Patient Liaison Committee of the British Pain Society and this brings her into contact with other voluntary organisations supporting and representing those living with back pain

- She represents patients' views through a number of other avenues and actively seeks to consult BackCare members by email and telephone in order to do this most effectively

- As a GDG member she consulted the BackPain helpline volunteers (n=17 and the majority, n=15, have back pain) on their views for the consensus questionnaire. Her final vote was informed by these views but based on her wider experience.

Nevertheless the GDG suggest that future guideline developers consider recruiting two patient representatives especially where a person of Nia Taylor's experience cannot be recruited.

10.7   Comparing these recommendations with other findings

This section compares findings here with those of other recent systematic reviews and guidelines in LBP. A main difference is that many other documents classify LBP as follows:

- acute LBP is < six weeks duration

- subacute LBP is six weeks to three months duration

- chronic LBP is > three months duration.

These guidelines consider physiotherapy intervention and are intended for people with persistent LBP of at least six weeks duration (i.e., sub-acute and chronic). This is more clinically useful for physiotherapists because:

- 80-90% of people with LBP recover within 6 weeks without physiotherapy intervention.[98-103]

The European guidelines for the management of non-specific chronic LBP recommend:

- supervised exercise therapy as a first line management intervention.

They did not recommend any specific types of exercise but suggest that these may be best determined by the therapist in consultation with the patient.[104]

A review of RCTs of exercise programmes for the relief of chronic LBP (n=51) found that the highest quality RCTs (n=16) all supported exercise and that the following were likely to be included:

- strengthening exercise

- supervised exercise (Liddle et al. Pain 2004;107:176-190).

A recent Cochrane review on exercise therapy for the treatment of non-specific LBP found that exercise was slightly effective in reducing pain and improving function in adults.[105] For subacute LBP the evidence

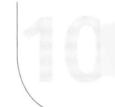

was less convincing although there is some evidence to support a graded activity programme to reduce absenteeism from work.[106] A sub-analysis of this review found that individually designed exercise programmes could reduce pain and increase function when they included the following types of exercise:

- supervised
- strengthening
- stretching.

It was also suggested that strategies to increase adherence to exercise programmes e.g., patient involvement were likely to be beneficial because high volume programmes are more effective than lower volume programmes.

In addition to the benefits discussed above exercise can also improve the wider aspects of fitness and health. The American College of Sports Medicine (ACSM) has published widely on exercise prescription and testing and their guidelines and their website is informative: **http://www.acsm.org//AM/Template.cfm?Section=Home_Page**

The details of the ACSM guidelines are outside the scope of this document but the guidance on resistance training, flexibility training, cardiorespiratory training and various aspects of exercise prescription are likely to be of interest to users of these guidelines.[107]

Therefore, in terms of main messages, this document appears to agree with other relevant literature i.e., patient involvement and exercise are common themes.

Nevertheless there are different emphases, for example, this document contains a detailed presentation of different exercise types. At the same time, the GDG recognise several other potential reasons for differences between this guideline and other comparable publications:

- all people with LBP of at least 6 weeks duration are included here but many reviews consider those with acute and chronic LBP separately
- research evidence here was only considered to be at level **Ib** where it was from *larger, higher* methodological quality RCTs, of robust statistical quality and these are tighter criteria than are commonly used
- RCTs on exercise, in combination with other physiotherapy interventions, were not considered here but might have been elsewhere
- different reviewers may have interpreted RCTs differently
- search strategies aimed at identifying all relevant RCTs may differ slightly and lead to a slightly different set of included RCTs.

10.8   Conclusion

This section has emphasised some important issues in the development of these guidelines for both guidelines' users and future guideline developers. Guidelines are fundamental to evidence based practice and it is hoped that the discussion here will assist future guideline developers.

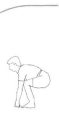

11 User feedback on these guidelines

Guidelines are intended as working documents and the CSP and the GDG welcome feedback from you, the users. For example, are the guidelines:

- useful to you as a clinician of any grade?
- useful to you as a person with persistent LBP?
- useful to you as a physiotherapy educator?
- useful to you as a physiotherapy student?
- well researched?
- well presented?
- applicable to you as a guidelines user outside the UK?

Has implementation of these guidelines been feasible?

Did the **audit pack** assist with implementing these guidelines?

Did the **quick reference guide** assist with implementing these guidelines?

Do you have any suggestions for improving future guidelines?

- If you are a chartered physiotherapist please feedback to us via the interactive CSP: www.interactivecsp.org.uk

The plan is to host a discussion under the 'discussion and exchange' part of the clinical effectiveness network.

- If you are not a chartered physiotherapist please direct your feedback to:

The Guidelines Team

Research and Clinical Effectiveness Unit

The Chartered Society of Physiotherapy,

14 Bedford Row,

London WC1R 4ED

Telephone: 020 7306 6666

Or email the corresponding author, Dr Anne Jackson at: **jacksona@csp.org.uk**

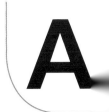

Appendix A

Scoping these guidelines

In April 2003 at the start of the guideline development process, a range of people were invited to discuss the scope of the guidelines.

The following people participated:
- Those who proposed back pain as a topic for physiotherapy guidelines
- Relevant clinical interest groups (i.e., those with an interest in pain, independent practice, acupuncture, manipulation, occupational health, the McKenzie approach, orthopaedic medicine and hydrotherapy)
- Two consultant physiotherapists
- A general practitioner
- A patient representative from BackCare.

At this initial meeting it was decided that the GDG should aim to include:
- Physiotherapists from regions throughout the UK and representing a mix of grades
- University educators and researchers
- Representatives from clinical interest groups
- A patient representative
- A policy maker
- Other health practitioners e.g., a psychologist, a general practitioner
- Input from other bodies e.g., occupational health, DSS, DoH
- Private practitioners
- CSP officers
- Experienced guideline developers.

The process of scoping the guidelines began at this initial meeting and was continued by the GDG at their first meeting in May 2003. The scope is given here.

1. All relevant health care settings.

2. Patients with the profile: between 18 and 65 years, with non-specific LBP, of three months or more duration (later adjusted to six weeks or more to include more literature) that may be recurrent.

3. Symptoms: the primary site of pain is the low back, leg pain may be present, there may be pain in other areas of the spine, there may be some non-progressive neurological deficit.

4. Exclusions: serious pathology, pregnancy, osteoporosis and spondylolysthesis.

5. Physiotherapy assessment is to include: a holistic and consistent approach, serious pathology (red flags) and psychosocial issues (yellow flags).

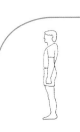

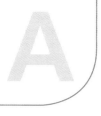

6. The range of physiotherapy interventions is to include: manual therapy, exercise, electrotherapy, hydrotherapy, acupuncture, cognitive approaches, biofeedback, relaxation, traction, functional restoration programmes, and education and advice.

7. Patient issues: e.g., compliance, adherence and empowerment, partnership with clinician, preference, choice, lifestyle changes.

8. Safety and adverse effects.

9. Management issues: e.g., patient pathways, discharge, onward referral.

10. Outcome measures.

Note that the scope for the range of interventions was narrowed later to exercise (including McKenzie exercise and hydrotherapy) and manual therapy (massage, mobilisation and manipulation). This was a pragmatic decision essentially to make the project manageable as described in the main document.

Appendix B

People involved in developing these guidelines

1. The guideline development group 2003 to 2006

Name	Post/dates of GDG membership	Speciality
*Panos Barlos BSc (Hons)PDD, Dphil, MCSP, LicAc	Research Fellow, School of Health and Rehabilitation, Keele University (October 2004 onwards)	Acupuncture
Katherine Deanne PhD, BSc	Systematic reviewer, CSP (October 2003-March 2004) Senior lecturer, Northumbria University (April 2004 onwards)	Systematic review
*Sarah Ferguson MCSP, MSc	Extended scope practitioner in orthopaedic spinal services, Royal United Hospital, Bath and Bath and NE Somerset PCT (September 2004 onwards)	Physiotherapy management of LBP
*Susan Greenhalgh MA, Grad Dip Phys, MCSP	Consultant physiotherapist, Bolton PCT (January 2005 onwards)	Biopsychosocial approach
Vicki Harding PhD, MSCP, MMACP	Research & superintendent physiotherapist, St Thomas' Hospital, London (January 2004 onwards)	Cognitive behavioural approach, pain management
*Dries Hettinga MSc	Systematic reviewer, CSP (June 2004 onwards)	Systematic review, sports science
Alison Hudson	Fundraising Manager, BackCare (April 2003 – September 2004)	The patient perspective
*Deirdre Hurley Osing BscPhysio, MappSc, PhD, MISCP, MCSP, MMACP	Lecturer, researcher, School of Physiotherapy and Performance Science, University of Dublin (Whole project)	Electrotherapy, Irish perspective
*Anne Jackson PhD, MSc, BA (Hons), MCSP, HT	Guidelines project manager, CSP (Whole project)	Guideline development methods, guideline writing, hydrotherapy
Jo Jordan MSc, MA, BSc(Hons)	Systematic reviewer, CSP (April 2003 to September 2004)	Systematic review
*Jennifer Klaber Moffett PhD, MSc, MCSP	Professor of rehabilitation & therapies, deputy director, Institute of Rehabilitation, University of Hull. (Whole project)	Exercise, cognitive behavioural therapy, patient education, guidelines development, research
*Denis Martin Dphil, MSc, BSc(Hons), MCSP	Principal Research Fellow, Sheffield Hallam University, Chair of the Pain Association Scotland. (Whole project)	Assessment of pain and its effects, Scottish perspective
*Stephen May MA, MACP	Lecturer, Sheffield Hallam University (October 2004 onwards)	McKenzie, exercise

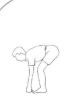

Name	Post/dates of GDG membership	Speciality
*Chris Mercer (Chair) MSc, MMACP, MCSP	Consultant physiotherapist, Worthing & Southlands Hospitals NHS Trust (Whole project)	Manipulation, exercise
*Jude Monteath MSc MCSP	Head of Therapies, Barnet & Chase Farm Proposed low back pain (Whole project)	NHS management and practice, ESP in orthopaedics and in pain management
*Lisa Roberts PhD, MCSP	Lecturer, University of Southampton and superintendent physiotherapist, Southampton University Hospitals Trust (January 2005 onwards)	Patient education, research, manual therapy
David Smith MCSP BSc(Hons) Dip Grad Phys	Superintendent physiotherapist, Fleet Community Hospital. Proposed low back pain (2003 to December 2004)	Extended Scope Practitioner (Spines)
*Nia Taylor MA, ACMA, BA(Hons)	Chief Exective, BackCare (October 2004 onwards)	The patient perspective
Alex Warne BSc(Hons)	Administrator, CSP (October 2004 to June 05)	Minutes of GDG meetings, organising meetings, assisting with the review process
Helen Whittaker BSc(Hons)	Administrator, CSP (April 2003 to October 2004)	Minutes of GDG meetings, organising meetings, assisting with the review process
Susan Williams BA(Hons.), MRSS	Administrator, CSP (June 2005 onwards)	Minutes of GDG, organising meetings, assisting with the review process, organising and recording the consensus process.
*Steve Woby PhD, BSc(Hons.)	Research Fellow, Physiotherapy Department, North Manchester General Hospital / Centre for Rehabilitation Science, University of Manchester. (Whole project)	Exercise, cognitive behavioural approach, guideline methods

* Indicates participation in the nominal group consensus process.

The nominal group involved in the consensus process 2005 to 2006

In addition to the GDG members, these people completed the first round consensus questionnaire in November 2005, participated in the on-line consensus conference in December 2005 and completed the second round consensus questionnaire in January 2006.

Name	Post	Speciality
Elaine Buchanan, MSc MCSP	Consultant Physiotherapist in Spinal Pain and Dysfunction at Nuffield Orthopaedic Centre, Oxford	Spinal pain and pain disability
Nadine Foster BSc (Hons), Dphil MSCP, PGCE	Senior Lecturer in Therapies, DoH Primary Care Career Scientist Primary Care Sciences Research Centre, Keele University, Staffordshire	Research and Evidence-Based Practice in lower back pain
Jackie Gracey, PhD, BSc(Hons), MCSP	Lecturer in Health Sciences, University of Ulster	Physiotherapy for LBP, ergonomics and occupational LBP
Nicola Hunter BSc, MCSP, MIOSH, RSP, CMIOSH	Founder and clinical director of RehabWorks Ltd, St Andrews Street South, Bury St Edmunds	Biopsychosocial rehabilitation and chronic musculoskeletal conditions
Jeremy Lewis PhD, MCSP, MAPA, MMACP, MMPA, MSc, PG Dip Sports Physiotherapy, PG Dip. Biomechanics	Research Physiotherapist, Consultant Physiotherapist (shoulders) St George's Hospital, Research Lead, Therapy Department, Chelsea and Westminster Hospital	Clinical research and evidence based practice relating to LBP
Christopher McCarthy, PhD, MCSP, MMACP	Research Physiotherapist, The University of Manchester Manchester Royal Infirmary	Diagnosis of types of low back pain
Ruth Sephton, MCSP, MACP, MSc	Consultant Musculoskeletal Physiotherapist (Spinal), Knowsley PCT	Physiotherapy for spinal conditions (clinical, teaching and research). Research of spinal triage services.
Kay Stevenson Mphil, Grad Dip Phys, MCSP	Consultant physiotherapist in musculoskeletal disease, University Hospital of North Staffordshire	Physiotherapy for spinal conditions
Jan Wroblewicz, MCSP, MSc, MMACP	Extended Scope Practitioner Superintendent Physiotherapist Royal Free Hospital Hampstead, London	Extended scope practitioner and manipulative therapist

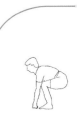

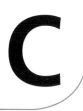

Appendix C

Literature search strategy

Literature searches were carried out to identify systematic reviews or randomised controlled trials published on low back pain and exercise/exercise therapy or hydrotherapy. Studies were limited to adults with chronic low back pain present for 6 weeks or more. Surgery and pregnancy were excluded.

Databases searched

AMED – Allied and Complementary Medicine (1985 to July 2005)

Cochrane Library – Cochrane Database of Systematic Review and The Database of Abstracts of Reviews of Effects search

EMBASE – Physical Medicine and Rehabilitation (1985 to June 2005)

HMIC – Health Management and Information Consortium database containing DH Data – the King's Fund database (1979 to July 2005) and HELMIS – the Health Management Information Service database (1984 to 1988)

MEDLINE - (1950 to July 2005)

SPORTDISCUS (1830 to July 2005)

PEDRO (1929 to July 2005)

PsycINFO (2003 to 2005 only, the GDG noted that this search was necessary in 2005 and earlier studies would have been identified from the systematic reviews).

Additional sources searched

The following sources were also searched for information:

Clinical Evidence

Guidelines Finder, via National Library for Health. National and international guidelines searched

National Research Register

CSP Library system (which includes details of books, documents, theses and dissertations, grey literature and CSP publications)

Bookdata

Search Strategies

Silverplatter webspirs was used to search AMED, MEDLINE, CINAHL and EMBASE: Rehabilitation and Physical Medicine. A combination of textwords and subject headings were used to find information.

1. Search strategies for MEDLINE

1.1   Subject search for MEDLINE

Exercise, including hydrotherapy terms (OR)

exp exercise therapy/

exp exercise/

group exercise.tw

stretching.tw

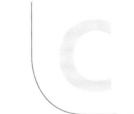

exertion.tw

exp hydrotherapy/

balneology/

AND

Low back pain terms (OR)

exp low back pain/

low* back pain.tw

chronic low* back.tw

1.2 Systematic review strategy for MEDLINE (Silverplatter)

1. meta-analyis.tw
2. meta analysis.tw
3. evidence-based-medicine/
4. guidelines/
5. exp practice-guidelines
6. data-synthesis/
7. data-extraction/
8. review in pt
9. published studies/
10. #1 or #2 pr #3 pr #4 or #5 or #6 or #7 or #8 or #9
11. comment in pt
12. letter in pt
13. editorial in pt
14. #11 or #12 or #13
15. (Subject terms)
16. #10 not #14
17. #15 and #16

1.3 Randomised controlled trial strategy for MEDLINE

1. exp randomised controlled trials
2. randomised-controlled trials/
3. random allocation.tw
4. double blind method/
5. single blind method/
6. clinical-trial in pt
7. exp clinical trials
8. clinical adj trial
9. single blind or double blind or treble blind or triple blind
10. single mask or double mask or treble mask or triple mask

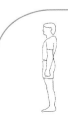

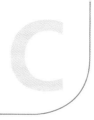

11. placebos/

12. randomly allocated.tw

13. allocated random.tw

14. #1 or #2 or #3 or #4 or #5 or #6 or #7 or #8 or #9 or #10 or #11 or #12 or #13

15. case report.tw

16. letter in pt

17. historical-article in pt

18. review-multicase in pt

19. #15 or #16 or #17 or #18

20 #14 not #19

21 subject terms

22 20 and 21

2. Search strategies for CINAHL (Cumulative Index to Nursing and Allied Health Literature)

2.1 Subject search for CINAHL

<u>Exercise terms, including hydrotherapy</u> (OR)

exp therapeutic exercise/

group exercise.tw

isokinetic exercises/

isometric exercises/

aquatic exercise.tw

pilates/ (from 2000)

stretching/

hydrotherapy/

aqua*.tw

AND

<u>Low Back Pain terms</u> (OR)

exp low back pain

chronic low* back pain.tw

lumbar vertebrae/

lumbar spine.tw

2.2 Randomised controlled trial strategy for CINAHL

1. clinical trials.tw

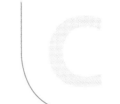

2. exp clinical trials/
3. clinical adj trial
4. single blind or double blind or treble blind or triple blind.tw
5. single mask or double mask or treble mask or triple mask.tw
6. randomi?ed control* trial*.tw
7. random assigment.tw
8. random* allocat*.tw
9. placebos/
10. quantitative studies/
11. allocat* random*.tw
12. #1 or #2 or #3 or #4 or #5 or #6 or #8 or #9 or #10 or #11
13. (Subject terms)
14. #12 and #13

2.3 Systematic review strategy for CINAHL

1. exp meta analysis
2. systematic review.tw or systematic overview.tw
3. exp literature review
4. medical practice evidence based/
5. professional practice evidence based/
6. evidence based practice/
7. exp practice guidelines/
8. guideline.tw
9. review.tw or overview.tw
10. literature review/
11. literature searching/
12. Cochrane.tw
13. Medline or medlars or embase or scisearch or psycinfo or pyschinfo or psyclit or psychlit
14. reference databases/
15. systematic review in dt
16. #1 or #2 or #3 or #4 or #5 or #6 or #7 or #8 or #9 or #10 or #11 or #12 or #13 or #14 or #15
17. (Subject terms)
18. #16 and #17

3. Search strategies for AMED (Allied and Complementary Medicine)

3.1 Subject terms for AMED

Exercise, including hydrotherapy terms (OR)

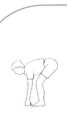

exercise/

exp exercise therapy/

exercise tolerance/

exp physical fitness/

physical activity.tw

strength*.tw

stretch*.tw

McKenzie.tw

aerobic*.tw

group exercise.tw

exp hydrotherapy/

aqua*

AND

Low back pain terms (OR)

exp low back pain

lumbar vertebrae/

lumbosacral region/

chronic low* back*.tw

3.2   Randomised controlled trial and systematic review search strategy

1. exp randomised controlled trial/
2. randomised controlled trial*.tw
3. random allocation.tw
4. randomisation.tw
5. placebos/
6. comparative study/
7. clinical trials.tw
8. double blind*.tw
9. single blind*.tw
10. treble blind*.tw
11. triple blind*.tw
12. systematic review.tw
13. systematic overview.tw
14. review.tw
15. guideline.tw
16. exp meta analysis/
17. meta-analysis.tw
18. metaanaly*.tw
19. #1 or #2 or #3 or #4 or #5 or #6 or #7 or #8 or #9 or #10 or #11 or #12 or #13 or #14 or #15 or #16 or #17 or #18

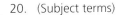

20. (Subject terms)
21. #19 and #20

4. Search strategy for EMBASE (Rehabilitation and Physical Medicine)

4.1 Subject search for EMBASE

<u>Exercise, including hydrotherapy terms</u> (OR)
exercise/
exercise-therapy/
physical fitness.tw
physical-activity/
aerobic exercise.tw
group exercise.tw
strength*.tw
stretch*.tw
McKenzie.tw
hydrotherapy/
balneotherapy/
aqua*.tw

<u>Low back pain terms</u> (OR)
low-back-pain/
low-back-pain-therapy/
low* back pain.tw
chronic low* back.tw
lumbar-spine/
lumbosacral-spine

4.2 Search strategy for EMBASE : Rehabilitation and Physical Medicine

1. Meta-analysis/
2. metaanlay*.tw
3. meta-analy*.tw
4. systematic review/
5. systematic overview.tw
6. quantitative overview.tw
7. quantitative review.tw
8. review/
9. short survey/
10. methodologic overview.tw

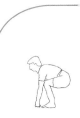

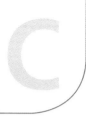

11. methodologic review.tw

12. collaborative overview.tw

13. collaborative review.tw

14. randomsed controlled trial/

15. random allocation.tw

16. randomly allocated.tw

17. randomisation.tw

18. clinical trial/

19. single blind procedure/

20. double blind procedure/

21. crossover procedure/

22. placebo/

23. single blind*.tw

24. double blind*.tw

25. prospective study/

26. practice guideline/

27. evidence based medicine/

28. clinical pathway/

29. #1 or #2 or #3 or #4 or #5 or #6 or #7 or #8 or #9 or #10 or #11 or #12 or #13 or #14 or #15 or #16 or #17 or #18 or #19 or #20 or #21 or #22 or #23 or #24 or #25 or #26 or #27 or #28

30. case study/

31. case report/

32. abstract report/

33. letter in dt

34. editorial in dt

35. #30 or #31 or #32 or #33 or #34

36. #29 not #35

37. (Subject terms)

38. #36 and #37

5 Search strategy for the Cochrane Library

5.1 Search terms

Cochrane reviews and Datatabase of Abstract of Reviews of Effects (DARE) searched

Exercise, including hydrotherapy terms (OR)

exercise/

exercise therapy/

exercise movement techniques/

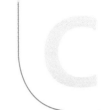

relaxation/
relaxation techniques/
physical fitness/
physical therapy techniques/
group exercise.tw
hydrotherapy/

AND

Low back pain terms (OR)
low back pain/
chronic low* back pain/
lumbar vertebrae/
lumbosacral region/
manipulation-spinal/

Key to search terms

pt = publication type
dt = document type
tw = textword
/ – subject heading

* = truncation symbol
? = variable character symbol

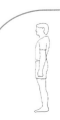

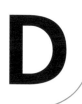

Appendix D

In tables 1 to 4 of this appendix, the data extracted from the RCTs are presented. These tables give detailed information to augment the evidence review (chapter 4). For further details readers are recommended to access the original papers. In general terms data included in these tables are relevant to the clinical questions asked in these guidelines.

Table 1 – gives some background of the interventions used in the RCTs and a description of the treatment, as presented in the original article.

Table 2 – shows the quality assessment of all included RCTs.

Tables 3a-3e – give the results of the included RCTs in terms of outcome:

- pain – table 3a
- function – table 3b
- psychological status – table 3c
- sick leave/return to work – table 3d
- costs – table 3e.

The baseline value, and the change over time, for each intervention group of each trial is given. Most RCTs have measured their outcomes at various points in time, in the tables these have been grouped in short term (less than 6 months post-intervention) and long term (6 months or more post-intervention). Improvements are always indicated with a + even where the actual value decreased over time. E.g., a decrease in 100 mm VAS score for pain is an improvement and thus this has been indicated with a + and a worsening of symptoms is indicated with a − 'Change over time' is displayed and not the 'post-score' since these guidelines address the question, 'which type of exercise is most effective'? The guideline development group considered that this question was best answered by comparing the **difference in change** i.e., **change in the intervention group** compared with the **change in the control or comparator group**. The 'difference in change' is expressed as an absolute value (change in the intervention group minus the change in the control or comparator group) and as a percentage of the average baseline value (which have been calculated by the reviewer and displayed in the baseline value column). This allows the reader to envisage the amount of extra improvement a person can expect by participating in a certain intervention:

+ indicates that the intervention of interest is superior to the control or comparator intervention

− indicates that the alternative intervention is more effective.

In addition to the judgment about the clinical relevance of this additional change that can be expected if the patient follows the intervention, it is also essential to consider the statistical significance of this value. If this difference in change was statistically significant, then the value has been marked with a * (significant at $p < 0.05$) or ** (significant at $p < 0.01$). NS indicates non-significant and NT means that the original article did not report statistics that tested this value.

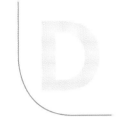

Example (fictional):

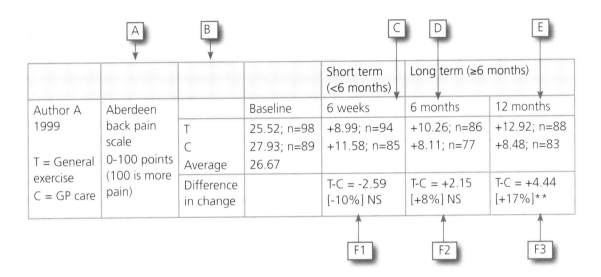

					Short term (<6 months)	Long term (≥6 months)	
			Baseline	6 weeks	6 months	12 months
Author A 1999	Aberdeen back pain scale 0-100 points (100 is more pain)	T	25.52; n=98	+8.99; n=94	+10.26; n=86	+12.92; n=88
		C	27.93; n=89	+11.58; n=85	+8.11; n=77	+8.48; n=83
T = General exercise		Average	26.67			
C = GP care		Difference in change		T-C = -2.59 [-10%] NS	T-C = +2.15 [+8%] NS	T-C = +4.44 [+17%]**

Author A conducted a RCT to compare the effectiveness of a **general exercise programme** with the effectiveness of **general practitioner (GP) care**. Effectiveness was measured using the Aberdeen back pain scale (A) and this scale was used at four points in time: baseline, 6 weeks, 6 months and 12 months.

The **baseline values for the treatment (T) group** and **control (C)** are given, in addition to **the average baseline value of the whole research population** (calculated by the reviewer) **(B)**. The change in these baseline values for the treatment and control group is presented at the 6 weeks point **(C)**, 6 months **(D)** and 12 months **(E)**. These change scores have a + if the change means an improvement in symptoms, or a − if the change is a worsening of symptoms.

The main value of interest is the **difference between the change in the treatment group and the change in the control group (F)**, this value is positive if the treatment group is superior **(F2 and F3)** or negative if the control treatment gave better results **(F1)**. The difference in change is given as an absolute value and as a percentage of the average baseline value. After this value the level of statistical significance is given: * for statistically significant at $p<0.05$, ** for statistically significant at $p<0.01$, NS for non significant values and NT if no relevant statistical test was reported.

The conclusion from this example would read as follows: A general exercise programme is similarly effective in reducing pain in the short term as GP care. A general exercise programme is similarly to more effective to GP care in reducing pain in the long term. The 17% **(F3)** is easiest to explain as follows: if the pain that a participant experiences at baseline is set to 100, than both treatments would result in the pain (and thus the score) to reduce over time (marked by the two +'s in box E), however following the general exercise programme would give an additional 17 points decrease in the long term. It is up to the patient and physiotherapist to decide if they find this 17% worthwhile (clinical relevance), but this 17% is a statistically significant additional decrease in pain.

Table 4 gives an overview of the RCTs that were excluded from this review and the reasons for exclusion. RCTs in the tables are alphabetically ranked on the first author's last name.

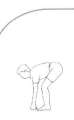

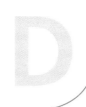

Table 1: Characteristics of physiotherapeutic methods examined in the included RCTs

Summaries are based on information in the papers and the style of language is that used by the original authors

RCT	Participants	Intervention	Duration	Expertise of therapist	Content	Outcome measures	Assessment
Callaghan 1994[59]	N=80 LBP >6 months CLBP	General exercise (8 sessions) vs General exercise (4 sessions) vs	4 or 8, 45 minute twice weekly sessions (ie over 2 or 4 weeks)	physio-therapists	**General exercise (8-sessions) [8 session Back rehabilitation group]:** Each session had an education element consisting of practical, demonstration lectures and an exercise element. These included sit-ups, wall slides, extension in lying, exercise bike, step-ups, standing – side flexion, push-ups (medicine ball), hip/knee rolling, flexion in lying, sit-ups (cross arms), rowing machine, arm pulleys, leg pulleys, skipping, wobble board, jogging, anatomy, posture, lifting, back video, hydrotherapy, dietician, discussion. The number of repeats of the exercises were specified at each session. At the end of the final session, the patients were given a home exercise programme. **General exercise (4-sessions) [4 session back rehabilitation group]:** Included sit-ups, wall slides, extension in lying, exercise bike, step-ups, standing – side flexion, push-ups (medicine ball), hip/knee rolling, flexion in lying, sit ups (cross arms), video programmes. Videos were used instead of practical demonstrations for all of the educational elements.[108] Although using a different medium the content did not differ from the 8-session group. Although the type and number of exercises were modified slightly to a regime with less emphasis on equipment and more compatible with home-based treatment, they exercised the same muscle groups and joints as the 8-session group. At the end the patients were given an exercise regime list based on the exercises performed in the back rehabilitation group and were instructed to perform these at home daily.	**Pain:** 0-100 VAS of pain **Other:** General well being, lumbar movements	Pre and post

RCT	Participants	Intervention	Duration	Expertise of therapist	Content	Outcome measures	Assessment
					Control group: Seen eight times. At initial session they were shown and asked to perform static abdominal exercises in crook lying. The physiotherapist followed a strictly structured protocol which ensured similar levels of attention as in the 8-session back rehabilitation group. Time was spent in the following way: re-evaluation of lumbar movements; performing a complete set of exercises; 5 min supine lying to 'rest' the back; lumbar movements rechecking; a general discussion of how they were coping with pain etc. and how they felt they were progressing. At the last session they were asked if they wished to join the back rehabilitation group.		
Donchin 1990[45]	N=142 At least three annual episodes of LBP. CLBP	Flexion strengthening vs Back School vs Untreated Control	Callisthenics: 45-min sessions, biweekly for 3 months Back School: four 90-min sessions over 2 weeks plus fifth session after 2 months	Physical education instructor physio-therapist	**Flexion strengthening [Callisthenics]:** Flexion and pelvic tilt exercises based on the Williams method aimed at strengthening the abdominal muscles, expanding spinal forward flexion, and rectifying general posture. **Back School:** Instruction in proper body mechanics as well in exercises for the back and abdominal muscles. Participants were encouraged to exercise at home on their own. **Control:** Untreated	**Pain:** Incidence of LBP episodes "painful months" **Function:** Oswestry LBP questionnaire **Other:** Trunk flexion and extension, muscle strength	Pre, post, 6 months follow-up

RCT	Participants	Intervention	Duration	Expertise of therapist	Content	Outcome measures	Assessment
Elnagger 1991[44]	N=56 LBP >3 months CLBP	Flexion (mobilising) exercises vs Extension (mobilising) exercises	14 30-minute sessions over 2 weeks	Physical therapist	**Both programmes:** Six sessions were supervised by a physical therapist; the remainder were conducted at home without supervision. For the home sessions the patients were provided with all the necessary instructions and illustrative figures to perform the exercises. The patients performed their exercise at a free pace and were encouraged to curtail their motion pattern. **Flexion mobilising [Flexion exercises]:** The number of times each exercise was performed per session varied according to the physical ability of the patient, but in general, each exercise was done 10 times, as suggested by Williams. Each exercise was done two or three sets per session; each set had five repetitions with 1 minute rest between sets. Each repetition was held for five counts before the patient returned to the starting position of the exercise. **Extension mobilising [Extension exercises]:** The protocol was derived from McKenzie's technique of therapy for the lumbar spine. The same procedure as in the flexion group was applied: two to three sets of exercises per session	**Pain:** Modified McGill Pain Questionnaire **Other:** Spinal mobility	Pre, post follow-up

RCT	Participants	Intervention	Duration	Expertise of therapist	Content	Outcome measures	Assessment
Gur 2003[65]	N = 75, adults with CLBP > 1-year	Laser + exercise vs l laser vs exercise	Laser applied 5x/week for 4 weeks. Exercise 2 sessions/day = 40 sessions for 4 weeks.	Laser: 2 physical therapist investigators. Exercise: initial session with physio-therapist	**Laser:** Application of the laser was external over a series of standardised fields designed to include the L4-L5 and L5-S1 apophyseal capsules, dorsolumbar fascia and interspinous ligaments, hamstrings and gastro-soleus muscles of which pain points were palpated from the low back to the foot. Stimulation time of four minutes was used for each point, producing energy of approx. 1J/cm2 (10.1cm2 energy density, 2.1kHz pulse frequency, 10W diode power, 4.2mW average power, 1cm2 surface) at each point. Approximately 30 min of total stimulation time was needed to cover the entire area of therapy for each patient. Standard technique was used with a gallium-arsenide laser (class IIIb Laser Product, Frank Line IR 30, Fysiomed, Belgium). **Exercise:** lumbar flexion and extension, knee flexion, hip adduction exercises and strength exercises of extremity muscle groups were given initially by a physiotherapist (1 session) then patients continued with them at home.	Pain VAS Schober Test Flexion and Lateral Flexion measures Roland Disability questionnaire (RDQ) (0-24 High = poor) Modified Oswestry Disability Questionnaire (MODQ) (high score = poor result)	Pre-therapy, Post-therapy (at one month).

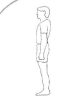

RCT	Participants	Intervention	Duration	Expertise of therapist	Content	Outcome measures	Assessment
Helmhout 2004[51]	N=81 (all male) non-specific LBP>12 weeks of continuous or recurrent (at least 3x/ week) LBP	High intensity extension strengthening training group (HIT) vs low intensity extension strengthening training group (LIT)	HIT: 10 sessions over a 12/52 period (2days/week in first 2 weeks then 1day/ week in weeks 3-12) LIT: not stated but impression given that it consisted of the same sessions as the HIT.	Trained physiotherapist	Each volunteer was given an intake test consisting of history taking by a sports physiotherapist, physical examination by a sports physician and pre-assessment of the isometric back strength by a human-movement scientist. HIT: progressive resistance training of the isolated lumbar extensor muscle groups. Initial training load set at approximately 35% of the maximal isometric back extension strength of the participant as measured in the first week. Goal of every training session was to perform 15-20 reps (weeks 1-2) or 10-15 reps (weeks 3-12) on the lower back machine equivalent to approx. 50% and 70% of the 1RM respectively. If the participant was able to perform a higher no. of reps, a 2.5kg weight was added in the next training session. On the other hand, if the participant was unable to perform the minimal no. of reps, the subsequent training load was lowered by 2.5kg. This training protocol was partly based on existing protocols and partly on the authors experiences. LIT: non-progressive, low-intensity resistance protocol uses. Throughout complete training period, training load set at no higher than 20% of max isometric strength as measured in the first week. The goal of every training session was to perform 15 (weeks 1-2) or 20 reps (weeks 3-4) on the lower back machine. The lowest training load on the machine was a fixed-weight of 2.5kg. In the authors opinion, resistance training at this level would not generated a significant physiological strength training stimulus. For both groups, training was carried out on a standard lower back machine (Lower Back ROM, Technogym, Italy) modified by applying a knee-lock system and a thigh-restraining belt to immobilize hips and thighs and isolate the lower back. In addition the oval-shaped "cam" was replaced with a circular "cam" as an earlier study found the circular shape better reflects the optimal load curve of healthy subjects.	Roland Disability Questionnaire (RDQ). Oswestry Questionnaire (OSW) Tampa scale for kinesiophobia (TSK) MOS 36-item Short Form Health Survey (SF-36). Net muscular torque (netMT) [calculated by subtracting the non muscular torque (passive test) from the functional torque (active test). Measured at the angles of 55 (full flexion) 40, 25, 10 and -5 (full extension) relative to the vertical].	Measures of outcomes taken: pre-randomisation. 1, 2 and 3 months post randomisation (treatment period) and at 6 and 9 months post randomisation (follow-up period).

RCT	Participants	Intervention	Duration	Expertise of therapist	Content	Outcome measures	Assessment
					Continued... For both groups flexion and extension of the lower back had to be executed in the participant's full ROM, movements had to be slow and controlled: moving in 2s from maximal flexion to maximal extension and returning from maximal extension to maximal flexion in 4s. During this movement, emphasis was put on the hollowing and flattening of the lumbar lordosis. Every training session was preceded by a 5-min all-body warm-up on arm/leg ergometer. The weight load used and no. or reps during each training session were recorded.		
Hemmila 1997[13] and 2002[14]	N=132 LBP >7 weeks SALBP CLBP	Physical mixed methods vs General exercise programme vs [Bone setting]	Physiotherapy: Ten 1-hour sessions over 6 weeks	Physiotherapists	**Physical mixed methods [Physiotherapy]:** Consisted of a combination of manual, thermal, and electrotherapy. The therapist was free to choose a suitable method within these categories and to use the facilities at their disposal: hot/cold packs, infrared heat, ultrasound, short wave diathermy, and transcutaneous electric nerve stimulation. In addition to massage, the therapist also employed specific mobilisations and manual traction according to the GP prescription, but no manipulations with impulse. Individual autostretching exercises were added if tightness of the pelvic or femoral muscles was noted at the initial examination. **General exercise [Home Exercise]:** Patients were taught a constant programme: to bend their low back rhythmically from side to side and back and forth as well as to rotate from side to side, ten times in each direction every 15 min, whenever sitting, standing, or lying still or at least before getting up in the morning and after lying down in the evening. The programme also included 10 sit-up, 10 arch-up, and 10 trunk rotation exercises twice a day.	**Pain:** 100mm VAS of pain Pain provocation score Pressure pain thresholds **Other:** Back mobility measures	Pre, post, 3 months, 6 months, 1 year follow up

RCT	Participants	Intervention	Duration	Expertise of therapist	Content	Outcome measures	Assessment
					Continued... The rotatory exercises were performed standing with feet apart, with small weights on both hands, rotating the upper body as far and as fast as possible. Autostretching exercises were added individually when appropriate. Repeated training sessions were booked only to ensure correct performance. **[Bone setting]:** The bone-setters were free to choose their own methods, which generally resembled chiropractic or osteopathy. Ostrobothnian bone-setting is, however, generally more gentle than it's academic counterparts. Their most popular method roughly resembles the sacral-push method for evaluating sacroiliac joint mobility described on pate 494 of the textbook by Bergmann et al 1993. It is, however, used to mobilize sacroiliac joints as well as spinal vertebrae from the lumbar to cervical region. The particular healers in this study, did not use the chiropractic adjustments described in standard textbooks, which are well known to many Finnish folk healers.		

RCT	Participants	Intervention	Duration	Expertise of therapist	Content	Outcome measures	Assessment
Johannsen 1995[57]	N=40 LBP >1 year CLBP	General exercise (endurance) vs General exercise (coordination)	1 hour session twice a week for 3 months (approx 12 sessions)	Physical therapist	**General exercise (endurance) [Endurance training]:** Each session started with 10 min warm up on a bicycle. Dynamic exercises emphasising muscle endurance were performed for the low back muscles, abdominal muscles, muscles around the shoulder girdle, and also hip abductors, hip adductors, and knee extensors. All movements were strictly controlled by strap fixation and physical therapist supervision. The patients were encouraged to do the greatest possible extension in the hips and spine, disregarding pain. Combined movements and rotations were not allowed. Each patient did as many repetitions of each exercise as possible up to 100, with 30 second pauses per 10 repetitions. As training was limited to 1 hour per training session, it was only possible to perform approximately four different exercises when 100 repetitions. After each session, 10 minutes of stretching of the trained muscle groups were performed using static stretching for 30 secs.

General exercise (coordination) [Coordination training]: Each session started with 10 min warming up on the floor, including jogging. Exercises emphasising coordination, balance, and stability were performed for the low back, shoulder and hip (figures in paper). Each patient did 40 repetitions of each exercise; it was possible to perform a wider variety of exercises than the endurance group. Combined movements and rotations were emphasised without fixation. All exercises were performed within a limited range of motion, respecting each patient's pain limits. After each session, 10 min of stretching of the trained muscle groups were performed using static stretching for 30 secs. | **Pain:** 0-5 point VAS **Disability:** Patient's rating of impairment (present or not) in 12 ADLs **Occupational:** Number of sick days **Other:** Analgesic consumption, overall assessment of effect. | Pre, post, 6 months follow-up |

RCT	Participants	Intervention	Duration	Expertise of therapist	Content	Outcome measures	Assessment
Jousset et al 2004[66]	N= 86, 18-50 yrs old, chronic low back pain	Functional restoration programme vs active individual physical therapy	Functional Restoration Programme (FRP) = 6 hours/ day, 5days/ week, for 5 weeks.	Active individual therapy (AIT) = 1 hour treatment sessions, 3 per week during 5 weeks. FRP = physiotherapist, occupational therapy, balneotherapy, physiatrist, psychologist. AIT = private practice physiotherapists.	**FRP:** The same programme was performed in 2 different rehabilitation centres. It was adjusted to each participant's capacity but always conducted as a group, sportslike activity. Frequent contacts between both teams ensured programme homogeneity. It included the following interventions: 1. warm-up stretching, proprioception: 9AM-10AM and 1.30PM – 2PM. Exercises included walking and running, "floor exercises", stretching of trunk muscles, balance exercises, and games. 2. Strengthening exercises: 10.15AM-11.15AM and 3.30PM – 4.15PM. Morning sessions consisted of isotonic training of all major muscular groups. Resistance was increased weekly starting according to the patient's progress. Afternoon sessions consisted of global strengthening exercises, supervised by a physiotherapist. The programme did not include isokinetic techniques. 3. Aerobic activities: 11.30AM-12.30PM. Activities included jogging and ball games. 4. Occupational therapy: 2PM-315PM. Sessions included training in flexibility, endurance and coordination, weight lifting and work simulation. 5. Endurance Training: 3.30PM-4.15PM. Jogging, stepping and cycling exercises were adapted to heart rate. 6. Balneotherapy: 4.30PM-5PM 7. Individual interventions: Patients met with the physiatrist who was the medical supervisor of the programme, every week and attended the weekly staff meeting twice during the programme. An appointment with the psychologist was scheduled during week 1 and if required, dietetic advice was provided.	1. Number of days of sick leave (if part-time, computed at half the total length) 2. trunk flexibility (fingertip-floor distance) 3. trunk strength (isometric contraction of the flexors and extensors as described by Ito et al and Biering-Sorensen. 4. Lifting capacity (progressive isoinertial lifting evaluation (PILE) test) – presented as % body weight. 5. Endurance (bicycle ergometers). 6. Pain (10cm VAS) during last 48 hours. 7. Impact on activities: French version of the Dallas Pain questionnaire (daily and work-leisure activities, anxiety-depression, social interest);	Before intervention, at 6 months

RCT	Participants	Intervention	Duration	Expertise of therapist	Content	Outcome measures	Assessment
					AIT: A precise intervention protocol was defined based on the recommendations of the French health accreditation and evaluation agency and on professional experience. The patient was free to chose his therapist from the group of available professionals. Treatment sessions included the teaching of a programme of exercises that the patient was to perform alone at home for 50 minutes on the 2 non-contact week-days. Each patient signed a written agreement to perform home exercises. During the programme only included active exercises. During the first 2 weeks, it was focused on flexibility, range of motion, and pain coping strategies. Strengthening exercises and functional training were then introduced. Patients were instructed to develop cardiorespiratory endurance by regular performance of sports activities. All patients were off work for the 5 weeks of the programme.	Quebec back pain disability scale. 8. psychological profile: hospital anxiety depression HAD) scale. 9 prescription medicine use noted.	
Kankaan-paa 1999[67]	N=59 LBP >3 months CLBP	General ex-ercise (active rehabilitation) vs Physi-cal agents (massage and thermal therapy)	Exercise: 24 1.5 hour sessions over 12 weeks Placebo: 4 sessions mas-sage & thermal therapy over 1st 4 weeks, passive therapy over final 4 weeks.	Physiothera-pist	**General exercise [Active rehabilitation]:** Groups of 4-5. The treatment included physical exercises with specific equipment, together with stretching and relaxation exercises. Behavioural support was provided by the physiotherapist, who described the "good prognosis" for LBP during the treatment sessions. Ergonomic advice was provided for each patient. Four specially designed training units[109] (lumbar flexion, lumbar extension, lateral flexion, and rotation) were used specifically to train trunk muscle function and coordination. The treatment was planned on the basis of baseline strength and mobility measurements.	**Pain:** Back pain in-tensity 100mm VAS **Function:** Pain and disability Index **Other:** Isoinertial back extension endurance test, electromyography	Pre, post, 6 months, 1 year follow up

RCT	Participants	Intervention	Duration	Expertise of therapist	Content	Outcome measures	Assessment
					The treatment began with very low loads for the first 4 weeks, with the object of improving mobility and especially of teaching coordination of the lumbar spine. The load was gradually increased so that between weeks 6 and 8, subjectively strenuous loading was applied for the first time. The load was further increased in a gradual and controlled manner up to 12 weeks. The range limitation ensured that the exercises were always performed in a painless range of motion. The subjects were instructed in back exercises that could be performed at home, and the importance of continuing these home exercises was strongly emphasised during the outpatient rehabilitation. **Physical agents [Placebo]:** The treatment methods, medication dosages, and guidance of the subjects were selected and designed so that the efficacy of the treatment was assumed to be minor. Thermal therapy and massage are assumed to be ineffective in the treatment of LBP, because they are not mentioned in the United States Agency for Health Care Policy and Research treatment guidelines for LBP. Patients received thermal therapy and massage individually for first 4 weeks. Passive therapy was administered during the final 4 weeks.		

RCT	Participants	Intervention	Duration	Expertise of therapist	Content	Outcome measures	Assessment
Kendall 1968[110]	N=47 'Long standing' LBP	Extension strengthening vs Flexion mobilising and strengthening vs Isometric exercises	Not specified	Physiotherapists	**Extension strengthening [Back extension exercises]:** Aims: To strengthen back extensor muscles. To correct posture deficiencies. To reach correct lifting techniques. Strengthening exercises: to be performed twice daily (6-12 times). Prone lying with hands clasped behind back; head and shoulder raising. Forehead rest prone lying; alternate hip extension. Yard lying; back extension with shoulder girdle retraction. Prone lying; head and shoulders raising with both hips extension. (Progress to neck rest, and then stretch to prone lying). Prone kneeling; alternate opposite arm and leg raising. Posture correction: In various positions including work situations and sleeping. Lifting techniques: With barbell and weights. With upturned stool. **Flexion mobilising and strengthening [Spinal mobilising and strengthening exercises]:** Aims: to increase ranges of motion in non-weight bearing positions; to strengthen supporting muscle groups, to correct posture deficiencies, to teach correct lifting techniques as a prophylactic measure. Mobilising exercises: all in maximum pain free range (6-12 repetitions). Crook lying, pelvic tilting. Heave grasp crook lying; both knees lowering from side to side with trunk rotation. Heave grasp crook lying; alternate hip updrawing with trunk side flexion (feet kept clear of plinth). Prone kneeling; back arching and hollowing. Prone kneeling; trunk rotation with alternate arm flinging. Prone kneeling; alternate trunk side flexion. Strengthening exercises: add one repetition at each visit. Lying: head and shoulder raising to place hands on knees.	**Pain:** Present severity of pain (3 point scale) Night pain (present or absent) Early morning pain (present or absent) Pain on forward flexion (present or absent) **Other:** Spinal flexion, spinal extension, straight leg raising.	Pre, 1 month, 3 months follow-up.

D

RCT	Participants	Intervention	Duration	Expertise of therapist	Content	Outcome measures	Assessment
					Neck rest crook lying; trunk flexion and rotation to touch opposite knee with elbow. Heave grasp crook lying; both hips flexion. Crook lying; pelvis raising (bridging). Prone lying; head and shoulders raising. Prone lying; alternate hip extension. The above exercises to be performed twice daily. Posture correction: in various positions, including work situation and sleeping posture. Lifting techniques: using bar bells with weights; using up turned stool. **Isometric exercises:** Aims: Correction of abnormal forward pelvic tilting lumbar lordosis. Strengthen abdominal and trunk muscles. Exercises: Crook lying (lying on the back with knees bent), contract the abdominal and pelvic floor and hip adductor muscles and hold the position for as long as possible, breathing normally. Standing, contract the abdominal and pelvic floor and hip adductor muscles and hold the position for as long as possible. Repeat both exercises 12 times, 3 times a day, and to repeat standing in the position as often as possible during the day. General advice on correction of posture, including work situations, sleeping and sitting.		

RCT	Participants	Intervention	Duration	Expertise of therapist	Content	Outcome measures	Assessment
Klaber Moffett 1999[58]	N=187 LBP >4 weeks, <6 months SALBP CLBP	General Exercises vs GP care	Exercise: Eight 1-hour sessions over 4 weeks	Physiotherapist	**General Exercise:** 10 participants in each class. The programme was similar to the Oxford fitness programme(78) and included stretching exercises, low impact aerobic exercises, and strengthening exercises aimed at all the main muscle groups. The overall aim was to encourage normal movement of the spine. No special equipment was needed. Participants were discouraged from viewing themselves as invalids and from following the precept of "Let pain be your guide" They were encouraged to improve their individual record and were selectively rewarded with attention and praise. Although partly based on a traditional physiotherapy approach, the programme used cognitive-behavioural principles. One simple educational message encouraging self-reliance was delivered at each class. Participants were told that they should regard the classes as a stepping-stone to increasing their own levels of activity. **GP care:** Patients allocated to the control group continued under the care of their doctor and in some cases were referred to physiotherapy as usual. No attempt was made to regulate the treatment they received, but it was recorded.	**Pain:** Pain diaries **Function:** Roland back pain disability questionnaire **Other:** EuroQoL health index (EQ-5D), fear and avoidance beliefs questionnaire	Pre, post, 6 months, 1 year follow up

RCT	Participants	Intervention	Duration	Expertise of therapist	Content	Outcome measures	Assessment
Koum antakis 2005 [49]	N=55, Non-specific low back pain – history of recurrent LBP (repeated pain episodes in past year collectively lasting <6 months, but onset of current episode > 6 weeks)	Stabilisation-enhanced general exercise group vs general exercise group	Class duration 45-60 minutes, twice per week for 8 weeks. Plus advice to do same exercises at home for maximum of 30 mins, 3x/week.	Senior clinical physical therapist (8yrs experience who had attended specialized stabilisation exercise seminars and applied them for approx. 1 year before trail initiation).	Both programmes included a warm-up period (stretching exercises and stationary bicycle for 10-15 mins). **Stability-enhanced group:** First session performed on individual basis lasting 30-45 mins. In this session, subjects were given individual leaflets to take home illustrating the anatomy of the local stabilising muscles, with written, clear instructions on how to preferentially activate these muscles. Briefly, low-load activation f the local stabilising muscles was initially administered, with no movement and in minimally loading positions (4-point kneeling, supine lying, sitting, standing).	**Pain report:** Short-Form McGill Pain Questionnaire (SF-MPQ) Pain VAS B (pain intensity over the past week on average) Pain VAS C (pain intensity over the past month on average)	

RCT	Participants	Intervention	Duration	Expertise of therapist	Content	Outcome measures	Assessment
			Due to a study showing that patients with subacute and chronic LBP activate their paraspinal muscles at about 30% of their maximum activation level during the performance of stabilisation exercises and at about 60% to 70% during the performance of muscle force exercises (trunk and leg extensions in prone), the authors set the pure total exercise time for the general exercise-only group		Progressively, the holding time and then the no. of contractions were increased in those positions up to 10 contraction reps x 10 second duration each (weeks 1-2). The clinical measure used to ensure correct activation of the transverses abdominis muscle was to observe a slight drawing-in maneuver of the lower part of the anterior abdominal wall below the umbilical level, consistent with the action of this muscle. In addition, a bulging action of the multifidus muscle should have been felt under the clinical physical therapist's fingers when they were placed on either side of the spinous processes of the L4 and L5 vertebral levels, directly over the belly of this muscle. Various facilitation techniques were used throughout the programme to draw subjects' attention to the specific nature of the desired muscle contractions (tactile, pressure, auditory, use of pelvic floor muscles) and subjects were made aware of and told to avoid several incorrect muscle activation strategies. Integration with dynamic function through incorporation of the stabilising muscles' co-contraction into light functional tasks was advised as soon as the specific pattern of co-activation was achieved in the minimally loading positions and the subjects could perform 10 x 10second contractions (weeks 3-5). Heavier-load functional tasks with exercises similar to those performed by the subjects who performed general exercise only were progressively introduced in the last 3 weeks of the programme.		

103

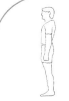

RCT	Participants	Intervention	Duration	Expertise of therapist	Content	Outcome measures	Assessment
			(99mins, 10seconds) to about half to that of the stabilisation-enhanced group (180 mins, 40 secs). This approach was followed to attempt to balance the groups with respect to the amount of estimated total force output of the trunk muscles targeted by the exercises.		**General Exercise group:** Exercises activating the extensor and flexor muscle groups were administered. Because muscle contraction occurring with exercise imposes extra loading on the spinal tissues, the general exercises were selected on the basis of maximizing the contraction benefit/spinal-loading ratio, according to recommendations provided from recent experimental studies. Eight exercise levels or progressively increasing difficulty were provided for both groups, if subjects were able to progress each week to a new level, based of graded exposure exercise principles. If this was not feasible for some subjects, they remained at the same exercise level. Subjects were seen in exercise groups (stabilisation-enhanced group 5-7 participants; general exercise group up to 10 participants). Subjects were required to keep an exercise diary monitoring home adherence. The clinical physical therapist monitored class adherence.	**Disability report:** Roland-Morris Disability Questionnaire (RMDQ) **Pain beliefs:** Fear of movement/re-injury measured with the Tampa Scale of Kinesiophobia scale Pain self-efficacy beliefs measured using the Pain Self-Efficacy Questionnaire. Pain locus of control Scale	
Ku-ukkanen 2000[60]	N=90 'Subacute' LBP, majority had LBP >3 months at 1st assessment SALBP CLBP	General exercise vs Untreated Control vs [Intensive training]	Mean of 3.5 sessions per week for 3 months	Not specified	**General exercise [Home exercise]:** The goals of the exercise programme were to increase the strength and endurance of trunk and lower extremity musculature, to improve body awareness, to promote dynamic stability and to control posture in order to diminish axial load and discal pressure, to decrease pain, and ultimately, to educate participants in the use of physical exercises for coping with the deconditioning syndrome. The exercise programme consisted of three monthly stages.	**Pain:** Borg scale (0-11) of back pain intensity and test pain intensity **Function:** Oswestry Index **Other:** postural sway, muscle strength, body mass index, dynamic extension and flexion, trunk endurance.	Pre, post, 3 months 9 months follow up

RCT	Participants	Intervention	Duration	Expertise of therapist	Content	Outcome measures	Assessment
					At the beginning of the latter two stages of the programme, the resistance levels of the various exercises were graduated. In addition, exercise performance was controlled weekly in terms of exercise technique and the number of repetitions performed for each exercise. Balance and co-ordination exercises were also included in the warm-up and cool-down portions of the programme. Strength exercises in 3-4 sets of 7-10 repetitions at 60-80% of 10RM (ten repetitions maximum). Endurance exercises in 3-4 sets of 15-20 repetitions at 30-40% of 10RM. The home exercise programme used no extra equipment to perform the exercises. (Diagrams of exercises available in paper). **Untreated Control:** Did not follow any prescribed training programme. [Intensive training]: This group were excluded from our considerations, as the patients were not randomly assigned to this group.		
Manniche 1988[111]	N=105 LBP >1 year CLBP	Extension mobilising and strengthening (high intensity) vs Extension mobilising and strengthening (low intensity) vs Physical mixed methods	30 sessions over 3 months Intensive back strengthening = 1.5 hour sessions; lower intensity back strengthening = 45 min sessions; Thermotherapy etc = 1 hour sessions	Physiotherapists	**Extension mobilising and strengthening (high intensity) [Intensive back strengthening]:** 1.Trunk lifting – prone on couch, hips at the edge, upper part of body free, but supported by the hands against the floor. Strap fixation over the calves. With hands on forehead, trunk is lifted to the greatest possible extension in the hips and spine, if necessary starting with support from the physiotherapist.2. Leg lifting – standing by the end of the couch, leaning over to a prone position, with the hips against the edge in 90° flexion, knees 45°, and feet on the floor. Strap fixation over the chest. Knee straightening and leg lifting bilaterally to greatest possible extension of hips and spine, again with support from physiotherapist if necessary.	**Pain:** 11 point box scales for current pain, worst pain in last two weeks, average level of pain for last two weeks. **Disability:** 15 ADL questionnaire **Other:** Back endurance, back mobility, analgesic use.	Pre, post, 3 months, 1 year follow-up

RCT	Participants	Intervention	Duration	Expertise of therapist	Content	Outcome measures	Assessment
					3. Pull to neck – sitting on a stool with the arms straight and abducted over the head and hands grasping a weight lever (pulley device). Against submaximal resistance the lever is pulled down behind the neck and shoulders. Before starting the three exercises the patient is offered a hot pack for 15 min. Each exercise is done in a series of 10 attempts, with 1 min rest in between. Exercise 1 is done 50 times, followed by exercise 2, 50 times, and so on. The training cycle is performed twice, interrupted by rest with a hot pack for 15 min. **Extension mobilising and strengthening (low intensity) [Lower intensity back strengthening]:** The exercises are done exactly the same way as above except that the exercises are repeated only 20 times. The dosage is therefore one-fifth of the intensive programme. **Physical mixed methods:** Applications of hot compresses and massage of back and gluteal muscles in combination with mainly isometric exercises for the lumbar spine; 1 (prone) isometric back extension, 2 (supine) crooklying (knees flexed, feet flat on couch) and isometric abdominal contraction, 3 (supine) crooklying and sit-up exercise, 4 (supine) maximal curl-up exercise, knees to shoulders. The exercises were repeated 10 times each within the limits of pain.		

D

RCT	Participants	Intervention	Duration	Expertise of therapist	Content	Outcome measures	Assessment
Manniche 1991[47]	N = 105, adults with chronic LBP (with or without radiation) >6 months or with 3 or more episode of acute pain within 6 months	Intensive back strengthening programme (C) vs modified back strengthening programme (B) vs alternative treatment (A)	**Group (C):** 1.5hr treatment, 30 sessions over a 3 month period as for Group (B) **Group (B):** 45min treatment, 30 sessions over a 3 month period (3x/week for 1st month, 2x/week for 2nd and 3rd month) **Group (A):** 1hr treatment, 8 sessions in 1 month	4 physical therapists	**Group (C):** 1. Trunk lifting (top half of body off end of couch, legs strapped down over calves, hands on forehead – lifting top half of body from floor to fully extended position). 2. Leg lifting (top half of body lying prone on couch fixed with strap over thoracic, hips at 90 deg, knees at 45 deg flexion, strap around knees to keep legs together – lifting both legs straight and off floor to greatest extension in hips and spine). Patient given support by physical therapist for both these exercises if necessary. 3. Pull to neck (sitting on stool, arms abducted and straight over head, hands grasping weight lever (pulley device), lever pulled down against submaximal resistance behind neck and shoulders). Before exercise programme starts, patient offered a hot pack for lower back for 15 min. Following this, each of the 3 exercises done in sequence as above. Each exercise done in a series of 10 attempts with 1 min rest between attempts. The first exercise is done 50 times, then the 2nd 50 time and finally the 3rd 50 times. The training cycle is performed twice but interrupted by rest with hot packing for 15min. In this way, each of the 3 exercises is done 100 times in the back programme. Participants train in teams of 4-5, where 2 physical therapists attended the training with help and instructions. Large movement fluctuation were attempted in all exercises and patients were helped in the last part of the movement track. Movements were not forced but executed as guided active movement. It was emphasized that exercises be performed at a dynamic but controlled pace.	Low Back Pain Rating Scale (0-100) consisted of subscales: pain (0-30), disability (0-30), physical impairment (0-40). Latter subscale was made up of objective tests (back endurance, schober's modified test, patients mobility, and use of analgesics). Qualitative Assessment: subjective marker rated very satisfactory, satisfactory (little discomfort), acceptable (some discomfort), unchanged, aggravated. Only the satisfactory and very satisfactory evaluations were considered as an acceptable outcome	Post-randomisation, 3 and 6 months and 1 year post-randomisation

RCT	Participants	Intervention	Duration	Expertise of therapist	Content	Outcome measures	Assessment
					The physical therapists realized that the exercises for many patients were associated with great strain and often elicited tension or pain over the lumbar region. However, if the exercises elicited or aggravated pain in the lower limbs this was not accepted. Training sessions consistently ended with thorough stretching of the working muscle groups in order to relieve muscular tenderness and discomfort. In the beginning, the physically demanding training was graduated in such a way that the patients at the first session did each of 3 exercises 50 times, in the following sessions 60 times etc until during a maximum course of 2 weeks, they were using the full training. **Group (B):** the 3 exercises are done in exactly the same way as in group (C) except that each exercise is repeated only 20 times. The dosage is thus 1/5 of that in group (C). All other conditions for training are identical with those in group (C). **Group (A):** patients were treated with applications of hot compresses and massage of back and gluteal muscles in combination with a mild exercise programme with mainly isometric exercises for the lumbar spine: 1. prone, isometric back extension, 2. supine crook lying, isometric abdominal contraction, 3. supine crook lying, sit up exercise, 4. supine, maximal curl-up exercise, knees to shoulders. The four exercise were repeated 10 times.		

RCT	Participants	Intervention	Duration	Expertise of therapist	Content	Outcome measures	Assessment
Mannion 1999[56] and 2001[112]	N=148 LBP > 3 months CLBP	Physical mixed methods vs General exercise (devices) vs General exercise (aerobic)	Physiotherapy Half hour sessions Devices: 1-hour sessions 12 weeks Aerobics: 1 hour sessions	Physiotherapy: Physiotherapists Devices: Specially trained therapists Exercise: Exercise instructors	**Physical mixed methods [Physiotherapy]:** the usual modern physiotherapeutic treatment administered in the hospital spine unit for this type of patient. Sessions focused on improving the functional capacity of the patient and giving instructions on ergonomic principles. Isometric exercises were carried out, and exercises with Therabands and general strength-training devices were performed. In addition, patients were advised on home exercises and encouraged to perform them. At times other acute problems (not necessarily back related) represented a hindrance to the planned back therapy, required treatment with passive therapies such as ultrasound, electrotherapy (TENS), short-wave, or heat/cold treatment. Each therapist was allowed a certain amount of freedom to adopt what they considered to be the most appropriate treatment programme for the individual case, but was expected to follow the guidelines drawn up by a senior physiotherapist. **General exercise (with devices):** The David Back Clinic programme was used(67, 113) with groups of 2-3 patients. It is an active functional restoration programme, the key element of which comprises controlled, progressive exercises carried out on training devices within the patient's pain-free range of motion. The exercises applied Isoinertial loading to the lumbar spine in the sagittal, frontal, and horizontal planes, in accordance with the strength-generating capacity of the trunk muscles. Relative progression of the loading was applied throughout the rehabilitation period. Each session was preceded by a 5-10 min aerobic warm-up (cycling, stepping). Relaxation and stretching exercises were carried out before and after the exercises performed on each device.	**Pain:** 0-10 VAS for pain intensity (greatest pain and average pain over last 6 weeks). **Function:** Roland & Morris Questionnaire **Depression:** Modified Zung Questionnaire **Psychological:** Fear Avoidance Beliefs Questionnaire Modified Somatic Perception Questionnaire Back Beliefs Questionnaire **Other:** Lumbar spine range of motion, Coping strategy Questionnaire, Psychosocial Aspects of Work Questionnaire, patient satisfaction	Pre, post, 6 months follow up

RCT	Participants	Intervention	Duration	Expertise of therapist	Content	Outcome measures	Assessment
					General exercise (aerobic): Small group classes (12 patients max) that included stretching and aerobic and muscle toning exercises carried out to music with an appropriate tempo and rhythm to promote the desired level of exertion. The programme was compiled from a range of sources. It comprised of a 10-20 min warm-up involving whole body static stretching and low impact aerobic exercises followed by 30 min of specific exercises directed predominantly at the trunk and leg muscles. The number of repetitions was increased, and more difficult variations of the exercises were incorporated, as the patient's became more competent. The last 15 min consisted of cool-down and relaxation exercises.		
Martin 1986(46)	N=36 LBP >6 weeks SALBP CLBP	Mobilising and strengthening exercises vs Isometric exercises vs Placebo (attention control, detuned ultrasound and SWD)	Nine 20 min sessions over 3 weeks		All: Given a standard hospital handout on guidelines for back care. Flexion strengthening [Mobilising exercises]: The function of these was to mobilise the joints in the lumbar spine and strengthen the abdominal and back muscles. The physiotherapists supervised patients for 10 min of each session, and then instructed them to practice on their own for 10 min. Isometric exercises: The function of these was to strengthen the abdominal and pelvic floor muscles. The regime was based on the LIFE exercises of Hume, Kendal & Jenkins. The physiotherapists supervised patients for 10 min of each session, and then instructed them to practice on their own for 10 min. Placebo: Participants were given 10 min of detuned ultrasound followed by 10 min of detuned short wave diathermy. The therapists was present to administer the detuned ultrasound but left patients on their own during the detuned SWD treatment.	Pain: Hourly pain ratings 0-5 point scale Function: 12 ADL items each rated for difficulty in performing on 100mm VAS, and scores summated to 1200 point scale Other: Spinal mobility, muscle strength	Pre, post follow up

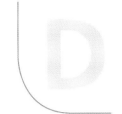

RCT	Participants	Intervention	Duration	Expertise of therapist	Content	Outcome measures	Assessment
McIlveen 1998[72]	N=109 LBP >3 months CLBP	Group hydro-therapy vs Wait List Control	8, 60-min sessions over 4 weeks	Pool volunteers with additional training in delivering the exercises	**Hydrotherapy**: 20 spinal exercises, 10 repetitions of each per session. Walk in water, forwards, backwards and sideways. Marching on the spot. Holding the rail and bobbing down in the water, bringing both knees up to the chest. Lunging to right and left keeping spine upright. Swinging legs forwards and backwards, and to the side. Rocking pelvis in the sagittal and frontal planes. Extension and flexion of whole spine. Lying on back: bicycling the legs vigorously; straight legs brought apart and together; each leg brought down towards the bottom of the pool alternately; and swing straight legs held together in the frontal plane. Rotate trunk. With a kickboard held in both hands: push and pull the kickboard down into water and pull up as hard as possible. With hand paddles on each hand: push the hands down past hips and behind, and then reverse movement and pull them up; with palms facing take the arms apart to side of body and then push together. (More details are available in paper). If a patient missed a session, an extra one was arranged. Any patient who missed more than one session was withdrawn from the study. **Wait List**: Untreated during the 4 week waiting period. **Both groups**: were reminded not to start any other treatment, medication or exercise programme for their LBP during the experimental period.	**Pain**: McGill Pain Questionnaire **Function**: Oswestry Low Back Pain Functional Disability Questionnaire **Other**: Lumbar flexion and extension, straight leg raise, tendon reflex grading, strength grading, light touch sensation	Pre, post follow up

RCT	Participants	Intervention	Duration	Expertise of therapist	Content	Outcome measures	Assessment
Petersen 2002[48]	N=260 LBP >8 weeks SALBP CLBP	Intensive strengthening vs McKenzie therapy	Intensive strengthening: A maximum of 15, 60-90 min sessions over 8 weeks McKenzie: Initial assessment and treatment 1 hour, subsequent sessions 30 min, intervals between sessions at discretion of therapist, maximum 15 sessions over 8 weeks Treatment could be stopped sooner if patients became asymptomatic	Physical therapists; All 7 McKenzie therapists had performed courses A-D arranged by McKenzie Institute International, 6 of whom passed credential exams during the period of this study.	**Intensive strengthening:** Groups of 6 patients under guidance of physical therapist. Sessions began with 5-10 min on stationary bike. This was followed by low-intensity, warm-up exercises for approx 10 min, comprising 10 repetitions of low resistance exercises for lumbopelvic muscles in flexion, extension, and rotation. After that, an intensive dynamic back strengthening training programme was performed in flexion and extension. It has been described in detail elsewhere. Four strengthening exercises were performed in a series of 10 repetitions with a 1-min rest between the series. The number of repetitions was graded individually. The initial dosage typically was 50 repetitions, whereas the dosage during the treatment period was gradually increased to 100 repetitions. At the conclusion of each session, the patients performed 10 min of stretching exercises for the trunk and hip muscles. **McKenzie therapy:** McKenzie treatment was planned individually according to the principles described by McKenzie. In short, treatment consisted of self-mobilising repeated movements or sustained positions performed in specific movement directions, the application of manual overpressure, and/or mobilisation by the therapist. **Both groups** were instructed to continue exercises at home or at a fitness centre for a minimum of 2 months after completion of the treatments.	**Pain:** Manniche's Low Back Pain Rating Scale Back pain intensity (3 separate 11 box scales of LBP at the moment, the worst LBP in last 2 weeks, the average LBP over last 2 weeks) Leg pain intensity (calculated in similar manner). Back and leg pain scores were summated into a 60 point scale. **Function:** 15 ADL items **Occupational:** Return to work **Other:** Use of analgesics, patients perception of change in back-related quality of life, visits to GP for LBP	Pre, post, 2 months, 8 months follow up.

RCT	Participants	Intervention	Duration	Expertise of therapist	Content	Outcome measures	Assessment
Rasmus-sen-Barr 2003[71]	N=47, adults, LBP >6 weeks with or without radiation to knee	Stabilising training group (ST) vs manual therapy group (MT)	ST group: 45 minute session, once/week for 6 weeks. MT group: 45 min. treatment, once/week for 6 weeks		ST group: Patients were told how to activate and control their deep abdominal and lumbar multifidus (MF) muscles. The first phase was cognitive and the patients were taught how these muscles act as stabilizers for the lumbar spine. The importance of re-learning motor control of these muscles was underlined. The patients were taught how to activate the deep abdominal muscles together with relaxed breathing in different positions (supine crooked-lying, four-point kneeling, prone, sitting and standing). The activation of MF together with the deep abdominal muscles was also trained. The physiotherapist monitored the patient by palpating the lower abdominal quadrant for deep tensioning of the deep abdominal muscles and by palpating the MF at the painful level. A biopressure unit was used in the learning process. The exercises were gradually developed by applying low load to the muscles through the limbs in different positions. The patients were instructed in how to use contraction of the muscles during activities of daily living, and in situations that set off pain. They were encouraged to perform a training programme, designed to take 10-15 min at home each day. They kept a training diary to monitor compliance. During each session the physio monitored how well the patient was able to control the muscle activity and to perform the exercises. The patients were also taught basic ergonomics. MT group: Manual techniques (Evjenth and Hamberg 1998, Grieve 1988, Kaltenborn 1989) were used, based on findings from the physical examination.	Pain VAS (10cm) (0 = no pain) General health VAS (10cm) (0 = best health imaginable) Oswestry Low Back-Pain Questionnaire Disability Rating Index (measures perceived difficulty in performing 12 daily activities on VAS – 10cm, 0 = no difficulty) Satisfaction with treatment VAS (10cm)	Pre- and post-intervention, 3 months, 12 months

RCT	Participants	Intervention	Duration	Expertise of therapist	Content	Outcome measures	Assessment
					They could include a combination of muscle stretching, segmental traction, and soft tissue mobilisation and if needed mobilisation of stiff thoracic and upper lumbar segments. No manipulation was done. The patients were encouraged to go on with their usual activities or exercises (not controlled). None of these exercises included specific stabilising exercises. The patients were also taught basic ergonomics.		
Reilly 1989[69]	N=40 "Chronic lumbosacral strain", but duration not otherwise specified	Supervised general exercises vs Unsupervised general exercises	Four sessions per week for 6 months (96 sessions)	Strength and conditioning specialist	General Exercises: Participants were given a predesigned exercise programme, comprising flexibility, strength, and aerobic exercises. Proper periodisation of programme was designed and participants were asked to adhere to this schedule and to increase as much as they felt capable. Supervised: Participants were assigned a certified strength and conditioning specialist who could monitor and work with each subject individually for each session. Their training took place in health clubs equipped comparably to that of the independent exercise group. Unsupervised [independent]: Participants were given the names of three comparably equipped health clubs they could attend. Compliance was monitored by health club staff.	Pain: 0-100 VAS of pain Other: Body composition, aerobic fitness, strength measurements, number of relapses that required medical attention.	Pre, post follow up
Risch 1993[62]	N=54 'Chronic' LBP, range 1-26 years duration. CLBP	Extension mobilising and strengthening exercises vs Wait List control	Twice a week for 4 weeks, followed by once a week for 6 weeks (14 sessions over 10 weeks)	Registered physical therapists	Both groups: Isometric strength of the lumbar extensor muscles was measured at 7 joint angles within each subject's range of motion up to 72° with a MedX lumbar extension machine. Participants were seated with their knees positioned so that their femurs were parallel to the seat and secured in place with femur and thigh restraints to stabilise the pelvis	Pain: Pain subscale of The West Haven-Yale Multidimensional Pain Inventory (WHYMPI)	Pre, post follow up

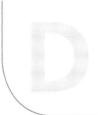

RCT	Participants	Intervention	Duration	Expertise of therapist	Content	Outcome measures	Assessment
					To begin each test, patients were locked into position at their most flexed position (between 48°–72°) and instructed to extend backwards slowly against the upper back pad. Once maximal tension had been achieved the patients were instructed to maintain a maximal contraction for 1–2 sec before relaxing, and resting for 10 sec, during which the next angle of measurement was set. The patients then completed a dynamic exercise through their range of motion with a weight load equal to one half of their peak isometric strength. They were instructed to complete as many repetitions as possible and then a 2nd isometric test was given, to enable a measure of muscular fatigue to be calculated. For the next two clinics patients were instructed in the proper training techniques. Instruction and training consisted of dynamic variable resistance exercise at a workload of one half the patient's peak isometric strength. When the patient exceeded 12 repetitions the torque was increased 5 ft-lb. When subjects returned for their 4th clinic visit they were again administered the 7-angle isometric strength test and then randomised to the treatment arms. Extension mobilising/ strengthening exercises: Variable resistance dynamic exercises. **Wait list control**: Placed on waiting list for 10 weeks and instructed to make no changes in their current lifestyle in terms of exercise training or other physical activities.	**Function**: Sickness Impact Profile **Other**: Mental Health Inventory, Exercise Locus of Control (Internal control), Peak isometric torque of lumbar exercises, WHYMPI positive and negative support subscales	

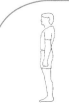

RCT	Participants	Intervention	Duration	Expertise of therapist	Content	Outcome measures	Assessment
Rittweger 2002[50]	N=60 Continuous LBP > 6 months or intermittent LBP >2 years CLBP	Extension strengthening vs Vibration exercises	18 sessions over 12 weeks (2 sessions per week during first 6 weeks and 1 session per week thereafter)	Not stated	**Extension strengthening [Isodynamic lumbar extension exercises]:** The participants performed exercises on a LE Mark1. After 1 min of warming up with lumbar extension (61Nm for women, 102Nm for the men), the participants rested for 1 min. Then they exercised, performing repetitive contraction cycles at a constant speed with a torque corresponding to 50% of the baseline maximum isometric values. As soon as the patient was capable of performing the exercises longer than 105 seconds (11 cycles), the load was increased in steps of 2.5kg. After completion of the lumbar extension exercise units, an additional resistance exercise of the abdominal and thigh muscles was performed (sit-ups and leg presses). **Vibration exercises:** These were performed on a Galileo2000(114). This consists of a platform that oscillates around a resting axis between the subject's feet. Hence, the amplitude can be controlled by adjusting the foot distance. As applied in the current study, the device has a maximum amplitude of 6mm, a vibration frequency set at 18Hz, and 4 minutes of duration for each exercise unit at the beginning, with 2 min of warm-up on the vibration platform (mere standing or squatting with small amplitude). The exercise duration was increased in steps to 7 min. During the exercise units, the patient performed slow movements of the hips and waist, with bending in the sagittal and frontal planes, and rotation in the horizontal plane. After 3 sessions, all the participants exercised at the maximum amplitude of 6mm. In a further progression of the programme, increasing weights up to 5kg were applied to the shoulders in subsequent sessions. (The complete exercise instructions are given in the paper).	**Pain:** 0-10 VAS pain scale. **Depression:** Allgemeine Depression Skala (ADS) **Other:** Pain related limitation, maximum isometric lumbar extension torque, range of motion in lumbar extension and flexion	Pre, post, 6 months follow up

RCT	Participants	Intervention	Duration	Expertise of therapist	Content	Outcome measures	Assessment
Shaugh-nessy 2004[70]	N=41, Chronic LBP >12 weeks	Lumbar stabilisation programme vs no intervention	10 exercise-training sessions over 10 weeks consisting of 2x1hour sessions in week 1, 2x30 minute sessions in week2, 1x30 minute session in weeks 3-6, and 1x30 minute session during week 8 and 10.	Chartered physiotherapist	Training programme was carried out as follows: 1. Subjects trained how to activate transverses abdominus and multifidus muscles. Facilitation strategies utilized by the physio included visualization techniques, verbal instruction, manual palpation and education using illustrations. Strength of contraction, monitored using a pressure biofeedback unit, was restricted to low levels compared to maximum voluntary contraction. 2. Training commenced in a low-load non-functional position (prone lying, 4-point kneeling, supine lying with flexed knees). Substitution strategies such as raising the rib cage, external oblique over activity or breath holding were avoided. 3. Holding time for exercises was gradually increased up to 10 contractions x 10second holds. 4. Once subjects were able to perform sustained contractions in low-load postures, the regime was progressed by adding leverage through limb movement. 5. Subjects performed a daily maintenance exercise programme at home in between exercise sessions with the physiotherapist. Subjects' performance of this programme was facilitated by means of written material (using physio Tools software).	Oswestry Disability Questionnaire Roland Morris Disability Questionnaire SF-36	Baseline and at 10 weeks for both groups.
Snook 1998[61]	N=85 'Persistent' LBP – mean duration 16.75 years CLBP	General exercise vs Avoidance of early morning lumbar flexion	Approximately 45 minutes training with instructions to continue programme at home.	Exercise: physical therapist Avoidance: the experimental investigator (Snook)	General Exercise: Described as a sham treatment consisting of 6 commonly prescribed exercises; pelvic tilt, modified sit-up, double knee to chest, hamstring stretch, side leg raise, and cat and camel. Each participant was also given written instructions and a videotape demonstrating the exercises.	Pain: mean pain intensity 0-10 scale Mean pain (days) Function: Mean Disability (days) Mean impairment (days)	Pre, post, and after cross-over follow-up

RCT	Participants	Intervention	Duration	Expertise of therapist	Content	Outcome measures	Assessment
					Avoidance of early morning lumbar flexion: Instruction in the control of early morning lumbar flexion. After a brief description of internal disc disruption, subjects were told that the first two hours after rising were the most important time of day to protect and maintain a straight back. Getting out of bed without bending the back was demonstrated. After rising to a standing position, subjects were told not to bend, squat, or sit for the first two hours. Standing and walking were permissible. Each subject was given a back scratcher to assist in raising the toilet cover or seat. A urinal was given to female subjects for urinating in a standing position. A reacher was provided for picking up objects from the floor. Subjects were told that after 2 hours, sitting, squatting, or kneeling with a straight back was permissible, but that actual bending should be avoided. After 4 hours, moderate activity with slight bending was allowed. After 6 hours, subjects were told, usual activities were allowed, but extreme bending should be avoided. The difficulties in complying with this schedule were discussed with each subject. Advice was given for shaving, showering, eating, cleaning teeth, getting dressed, and having bowel movements. Changing the daily routine was suggested so that bending activities or heavier physical activities could be performed later in the day or in the evening when the back is less vulnerable. Subjects told to plan ahead, to arrange their clothes and toilet articles in the evening so early morning bending would not be necessary. The possibility of getting up earlier was suggested.	Other: Mean medication	

RCT	Participants	Intervention	Duration	Expertise of therapist	Content	Outcome measures	Assessment
					It was emphasised that partial compliance with the schedule was better than no compliance. Subjects were asked to record the time they were able to stand every morning without bending, squatting, or sitting. A stopwatch was provided to assist in obtaining accurate times of compliance. Participants were also told not to expect an immediate reduction in pain, and that any improvement would not be noticed for several days or weeks.		
Storheim 2003[54]	N=93, non-specific low back pain sick-listed for 8-12 weeks	Exercise regime vs cognitive intervention vs control group	**Exercise group** 15 weeks with a minimum of 2x/week exercise sessions (preferably 3x/week) each session lasting for 1 hour. **Cognitive group:** 2 consultations offered each lasting 30-60 minutes. Then invited to telephone the specialist	Standard clinical examination by specialist in physical medicine. **Exercise group** Experienced physical therapists **Cognitive group** first appointment –specialist in physical medicine and physical therapist.	Exercise and cognitive groups underwent a standard clinical examination which consisted of a routine back examination, explanation of x-rays and CT-scans, and general encouragement to resume daily activities and work. Additionally answers to a questionnaire completed at inclusion were discussed with the patient. A report was sent to the GP and to the local National Insurance Office. **Exercise group:** patients were randomised into ongoing back training groups at a large physical therapy practice. Group training was a modification of The Norwegian Aerobic Fitness Model. This concept is based on both exercise physiology and ergonomic principles, and designed to increase overall fitness and functional capacity (CV, Strength – particularly in thighs, back-abdominal (incl transversus abdominal) and pelvic floor muscles, flexibility, body awareness and relaxation). The whole programme is accompanied by music. Modification of the training model for the patients with LBP are: - a physical therapist choreographed the programme and every training session was led by experienced physical therapists	Pain VAS x 2 - One for LBP and one for lower limb pain measuring greatest pain at present). Pain diary completed 3x/day for 7 days before and after treatment (2 VAS scales: how strong is your pain (sensory pain) and how distressing is your pain (affective pain)). Consumption of painkillers registered on 4 point scale (1=daily, 2 = weekly, 3 = less than every week, 4 = never).	

RCT	Participants	Intervention	Duration	Expertise of therapist	Content	Outcome measures	Assessment
			or the physical therapist for advice or consultations	Control group: GP	- focus on ergonomic principles and functional tasks - no pain focus - it is safe to move The physical therapy practice offered back training groups at different intensity levels. Patients started at the lowest level and increased the intensity by entering into more advanced classes. Subjects with the best progress were transferred to ordinary classes for healthy people outside the physical therapy practice, organized in accordance with the exercise model and by the same physical therapist responsible for the programme in the back training classes. Patients' attendance at the training classes was registered in training diaries kept in the physical therapy practice. **Cognitive intervention:** patients were assigned a new appointment at the outpatient clinic as soon as possible after the standard clinical examination. The following items were dealt with: - explanation of pain mechanisms - questionnaire completed at inclusion was discussed once more in-depth - functional examination with individual feedback and advice. - instruction in activation of deep stabilising muscles (transverses) and advice on how to use it actively in functional and demanding tasks of daily life. - instruction in the squat technique when lifting is required - how to cope with new attacks - reassure and emphasize that it is safe to move and to use the back without restriction. **Control group:** patients were treated by their GP and had no restrictions of treatments or referrals.	Roland Morris questionnaire Sick-listing Fear-avoidance beliefs evaluated using Waddell's Fear-Avoidance Belief Questionnaire (FABQ) Hopkins Symptom Checklist (HSCL-25) for emotional distress. SF-36 health survey for generic health status. Life satisfaction was estimated by Cantrils Ladder Scale.	

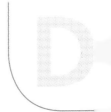

RCT	Participants	Intervention	Duration	Expertise of therapist	Content	Outcome measures	Assessment
Torsten-sen 1998[55]	N=208 LBP >8 weeks <52 weeks SALBP CLBP	General exercise vs Physical mixed methods vs Walking	36 one hour sessions over 12 weeks		**General exercise [Medical exercise therapy]:** This system of progressively graded exercises was developed by Holten. Their aim is to normalise function using specific exercises for mobilising hypomobile areas of the spine and by designing stabilising exercises for other parts. Given in groups (max 5 participants) under supervision of physiotherapist.. Each patient in the group has an individually designed exercise programme related to symptoms, clinical diagnosis, needs and expectations. Progressions for the exercises are made possible by the use of specially designed equipment such as the wall pulley, lateral pulley, angle bench, multipurpose bench, incline board, wall bar, deloading frame, dumbbells, and bar bells. In using this equipment the grading is a function of the starting position, resistance applied, range of motion, number and speed of repetitions, number of sets, and number of treatments during the week. Patients were given 7-9 different exercises. They performed 2-3 sets of 20-30 repetitions each with 30 seconds of rest between each set. Before doing the treatment patients performed a maximum test of each exercise, with 40 repetitions within defined parameters. Subtracting 20% of these 40 repetitions, the patient for treatment purposes does 32 repetitions in three sets with a 30 sec break between each set. The grading of the exercises makes it possible to exercise with no (or virtually no) pain. At least the pain should not increase during training.	**Pain:** Pain intensity 100mm VAS for back pain combined with pain intensity 100mm VAS for leg pain (200mm in total) **Function:** Oswestry Low Back Pain Disability Questionnaire **Occupational:** return to work **Costs:** Total costs **Other:** Satisfaction with treatment	Pre, 1 year follow-up

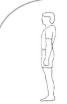

RCT	Participants	Intervention	Duration	Expertise of therapist	Content	Outcome measures	Assessment
					In the introductory phase exercise positions are selected to give the intervertebral disc a minimal pressure (i.e., standing and lying as compared with sitting). The patient has a 10-15 minute warm-up before the exercise programme. **Physical mixed methods [Conventional physiotherapy]:** *a combination of methods such as heat or cold, massage, stretching, different forms of electrotherapy, traction, and a few exercises on the treatment table. The physiotherapist could combine any of their methods available except for an intensive exercise programme.* **Walking [Self exercise]:** All patients in this group received information about self exercise by walking and the importance of activity for the back. The patients were encouraged to walk for 1 hour three times a week. Preferably there was to be 1 day of rest between each hour walking. The project leader phoned these participants every second week during the intervention period (6 contacts) to encourage compliance.		
Tritilanunt 2001[43]	N=72 LBP >3 months CLBP	General exercise (aerobic) vs Flexion mobilising	12 weeks	Not stated	**General exercise (aerobic):** Aerobic exercise, a series of 3 health education sessions including a group discussion, modelling, demonstration and self practice. **Flexion mobilising:** Included regular health education, postural and behavioural instruction and a lumbar flexion exercise programme. **Both groups:** Non-steroidal anti-inflammatory drugs were not used, but analgesics were administered in cases with moderate or sever back pain.	**Pain:** Pain 0-10 VAS Other: Resting pulse, blood pressure on lying, body weight, occupation, activity and serum for High Density Lipoprotein Cholesterol (HDL-C).	Pre, post follow-up

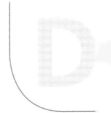

RCT	Participants	Intervention	Duration	Expertise of therapist	Content	Outcome measures	Assessment
Turner 1990[53]	N=96 LBP >=6 months CLBP	Operant Behavioural Vs Operant Behavioural + general exercise Vs General Exercise (control) Vs Waiting list control	Behavioural: Eight 2-hour sessions over 8 weeks Exercise: 10-20 min sessions five times a week	PhD-level	**Operant Behavioural:** (Fordyce) patient + spouse education on pain behaviours, reinforcement, communication training, behavioural goals **General aerobic exercise:** gradual and systematic increase of fast walking/slow jogging based on quota system (Fordyce). Progressing from 10 min to 20 min and from 60% to 70% estimated maximum heart rate. Patients were also instructed in the use of warm-up and cool-down stretches to perform each time they exercised. **Behavioural + exercise:** subjects received both treatments as described above. **Waitlist:** patients did not receive any treatment for 8 weeks	**Pain:** MPQ Pain Rating Index **Function/disability:** Sickness Impact Profile (Bergner, 1981) - patients + spouse; Pain Behaviour Checklist (Turk, 1985) patients + spouse; Observer ratings of pain - videotapes of set movement (Keefe, 1982) **Psychological:** Depression - The Centre for Epidemiologic Studies Depression Scale (Radloff, 1977) **Other:** Physical fitness - physical work capacity, strength, flexibility; Patient rating of treatment - satisfaction and helpfulness of treatment	Pre, post, 6-months, 12-months follow-up

RCT	Participants	Intervention	Duration	Expertise of therapist	Content	Outcome measures	Assessment
UK-BEAM 2005[63, 64]	N=1334 patients who consulted their GP for low back pain, all subjects had a score of 4 or more on the Roland Disability Question-naire	Best care vs. best care +exercise vs. best care + manipulation vs. best care + exercise + manipulation	Exercise: up to 8 sessions over 4-8 weeks and a refresher class at 12 weeks. Manipulation: up to 8 sessions over 12 weeks. Combined: 8 sessions of manipulation in first 6 weeks followed by 8 sessions of exercise in the next 6 weeks	Experiences	**Best care:** 'standard GP care' based on UK guidelines advising to continue normal activity and avoiding rest. Supported by the Back Book for patients and GP practices. **Exercise:** 'Back to Fitness' exercise programme, based on cognitive behavioural principles. Classes run in local community facilities with up to 10 participants. Session took 60 minutes. **Manipulation:** A MDT group developed a package of techniques as used in the UK by physiotherapists, osteopaths and chiropractors. Manipulation was conducted by the same therapists in either private or NHS setting and they could choose from the agreed range of techniques. Most patients got high velocity thrusts at least once. Sessions took 20 minutes. **Combined:** 8 sessions of manipulation followed by 8 sessions of exercise, as above described.	**Pain:** Von Korff scale **Function:** Roland Morris Disability Questionnaire, modified Von Korff scales **Psychological status:** back beliefs questionnaire, fear avoidance beliefs questionnaire.	Baseline, 3 months and 12 months follow up
Yoz-batiran 2004[68]	N=30, adults, CLBP > 3 months	Fitness group vs aquafitness group	3days/week for 4 weeks		Programme of **fitness group** consisted of warm-up and stretching followed by a circuit of 15 progressive exercises, and cool down with stretching and light aerobic exercise, according to the programme described by Frost et al 1995, 1998. The **aquafitness group** followed the same programme in a pool.	Pain VAS (10cm, 0 = no pain) Oswestry low back disability questionnaire (high score = high disability)	Pre- and post-treatment

RCT	Participants	Intervention	Duration	Expertise of therapist	Content	Outcome measures	Assessment
						Musculoskeletal fitness (dynamic sit-up, flexibility sit and reach test, motor fitness single leg balance test)	
						Anthropometry – body composition (skinfold, BMI, waist-to-hip ratio).	
						Aerobic fitness (12 min walk test)	
						Isometric extensor trunk endurance test (Sorensen test)	

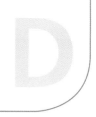

Table 2: Quality assessment of the RCTs

Adapted van Tulder Methodological Quality Criteria[10]

a   Treatment allocation: Was the treatment allocation concealed?

b   Were the groups similar at baseline regarding the most important prognostic indicators? (e.g., age, duration of complaints, value of main outcome measures)

c   Was the care provider blinded to the intervention?

d   Were co-interventions avoided or comparable?

e   Was the compliance rate (in each group) unlikely to cause bias?

f   Was the patient blinded to the intervention?

g   Was the outcome assessor blinded to the intervention?

h   Was the withdrawal / drop-out rate unlikely to cause bias?

i   Was the timing of the outcome assessments in both groups comparable?

j   Did the analysis include an intention-to-treat analysis?

The 10 items above have been used to calculate the 10-point score as mentioned in the guideline.

	a	b	c	d	e	f	g	h	i	j	Tot.
Callaghan 1994[59]	-	+	-	?	?	-	?	?	+	?	2/10
Donchin 1990[45]	+	+	-	-	-	-	-	+	+	+	5/10
Elnagger 1991[44]	+	+	-	-	-	-	+	-	+	+	5/10
Gur 2003[65]	-	+	-	?	+	-	+	+	+	-	5/10
Helmhout 2004[51]	+	-	-	-	-	-	+	-	+	-	3/10
Hemmila 1997[13] + 2002[14]	+	+	-	+	-	-	+	+	+	+	7/10
Johannsen 1995[57]	?	?	-	-	-	-	-	-	+	-	1/10
Jousset 2004[66]	?	+	-	-	+	-	-	+	+	-	4/10
Kankaanpaa 1999[67]	-	?	?	?	+	-	-	+	+	-	3/10
Kendall 1968[110]	?	-	-	-	-	-	-	+	+	-	2/10
Klaber Moffett 1999[58]	+	+	?	?	+	-	+	+	+	+	7/10
Koumantakis (phys ther) 2005[49]	+	+	-	?	+	-	+	+	+	+	7/10
Kuukkanen 2000[60]	-	+	?	?	+	?	?	+	+	-	4/10
Martin 1986[46]	-	-	-	-	-	-	-	-	+	-	1/10
Manniche 1988[111]	+	+	-	+	-	-	+	+	+	+	7/10
Manniche 1991[47]	-	?	-	-	-	-	+	-	+	-	2/10
Mannion 1999[56]+ 2001[112]	+	+	-	+	+	+	+	+	+	+	9/10
McIlveen 1998[72]	+	+	?	?	+	-	+	+	+	-	6/10
Petersen 2002[48]	+	+	?	?	+	-	-	+	+	+	6/10
Rasmussen-Barr 2003[71]	?	+	-	-	?	-	?	-	+	-	2/10
Reilly 1989[69]	-	-	-	?	?	-	-	+	+	+	2/10

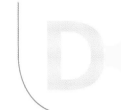

	a	b	c	d	e	f	g	h	i	j	tot.
Risch 1993[62]	-	+	-	-	-	-	-	+	+	+	4/10
Rittweger 2002[50]	?	+	?	?	+	-	-	+	+	-	4/10
Shaughnessy 2004[70]	?	+	-	?	-	-	?	-	+	-	2/10
Snook 1998[61]	-	+	-	-	+	+	+	+	?	+	6/10
Storheim 2003[54]	+	+	-	-	-	-	+	-	+	+	5/10
Torstensen 1998[55]	+	+	-	+	+	-	+	+	+	+	8/10
Tritilanunt 2001[43]	+	+	-	+	+	-	-	+	+	-	6/10
Turner 1990[53]	-	+	-	?	?	-	+	+	+	-	4/10
UK BEAM 2004[63, 64]	+	+	-	+	?	-	-	+	+	+	6/10
Yozbatiran 2004[68]	-	+	-	?	+	-	?	+	+	+	5/10

+ RCT has fulfilled criteria

- RCT has not fulfilled criteria

? It is unclear from the original text if the RCT has fulfilled the criteria

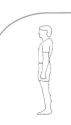

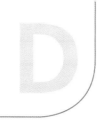

Table 3a: Main outcomes: Pain

RCT	Measure		Baseline	Short term (<6 months)	Long term (≥6 months)
Callaghan 1994[59] T1 = general exercises (8 sessions) T2 = general exercises (4 sessions) C = Control	Percentage change on 100 point VAS for pain		Baseline	Post intervention	
		T1	NA ;n=30	+53% ;n=30	
		T2	NA ;n=30	+47% ;n=30	
		C	NA ;n=20	0% ;n=20	
		Average	?		
		Difference in change		T1-T2= +6% NS T1-C= +53% *	
Donchin 1990[45] T1 = flexion strengthening T2 = back school C = untreated	Painful months in year following treatment (graph)		Baseline		12 months
		T1	NA		+4.5 n=46
		T2	NA		+7.3 n=46
		C	NA		+7.4 n=50
		Average	?		
		Difference in change			T1-C = +2.9 ** T1-T2 = +2.8 **
Elnagger 1991[44] T1 = flexion mobilising T2 = extension mobilising	Modified McGill Pain Questionnaire		Baseline	Post intervention	
		T1	15.9 n=28	+5.3; n=28	
		T2	14.1 n=28	+5.2; n=28	
		Average	15		
		Difference in change		T1-T2= +0.1 [+0.7%#] NS	

In 'change' column: + improvement, - worsening of symptoms
In 'difference in change' cell: * statistically significant at p<0.05, ** statistically significant at p<0.01, NS not significant, NT not tested, + intervention of interest is more effective than comparator, - intervention of interest is less effective than comparator

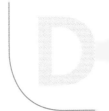

RCT	Measure		Baseline	Short term (<6 months)	Long term (≥6 months)
Gur 2003[65] T1 = laser + exercise T2 = exercise T3 = laser	Pain VAS (0-10)		Baseline	Post intervention	
		T1	6.2(2.1); n=25	+4.4; n=25	
		T2	6.5(1.6); n=25	+3.6; n=25	
		T3	6.1(1.9); n=25	+4.2; n=25	
		Average	6.3	6.3	
		Difference in change		T1-T2 = +0.8 [12.7%#] NS T1-T3 = +0.2 [3.2%#] NS	
Hemmila 1997[13] and 2002[14] T1 = physiotherapy T2 = home exercise C= bone setting	Pain VAS (0-100mm) (data from graph)		Baseline	6 weeks	3 months	6 months
		T1	43 ;n=34	+18 ;n=34	+17 ;n=34	+18 ;n=34
		T2	41 ;n=35	+11 ;n=35	+10 ;n=35	+11 ;n=35
		C	46 ;n=45	+16 ;n=45	+16 ;n=45	+21 ;n=45
		Average	44			
		Difference in change		T2-T1 = -7 [-15%#] NS T2-C = -5 [-11%#] NS	T2-T1 = -7 [-15%#] NS T2-C = -6 [-13%#] NS	T2-T1 = -7 [-15%#] NS T2-C = -10 [-22%#]*
Johannsen 1995[57] T1 = general endurance exercises T2= general coordination exercises	Sum of two pain scores on a 0-4 scale (sum of current pain and pain in past week) 0-8		Baseline	3 months	6 months
		T1	6; n=20	+3; n=13	+2; n=13
		T2	6; n=20	+1; n=14	+2; n=14
		Average	6		
		Difference in change		T1-T2 = +2 [+33%#] NS	T1-T2 = 0 [0%#] NS

RCT	Measure		Baseline	Short term (<6 months)	Long term (≥6 months)
Jousset et al 2004[66] T1 = Functional restoration programme T2 = active individual physical therapy	Pain during past 24hours (10cm VAS, 0 = no pain, 10 = maximal pain)		Baseline		6 months
		T1	5.0(2.2);n=42		+1.9 ;n=42
		T2	4.6(2.2);n=41		+0.6 ;n=41
		Average	4.8		
		Difference in change			T1-T2 = +1.3 [+27.1% #] NT
Kankaanpaa 1999[67] T = General exercise (active rehab) C = Physical agents (passive rehab)	Pain intensity 100mm VAS		Baseline	Post intervention	6 months / 12 months
		T	55.2; n=30	+19.7; n=30	+28.6; n=28 / +31.3; n=27
		C	47.0: n=24	+3.2; n=24	+3.6; n=22 / +1.9; n=22
		Average	51.1		
		Difference in change		T-C = +16.5 [+32%#] *	T-C = +25.0 [+49%#] ** / T-C = +29.4 [+58%#] **
Klaber Moffett 1999[58] T = General exercise C = GP care	Aberdeen back pain scale (0-100 points)		Baseline	6 weeks	6 months / 12 months
		T	27.93; n=98	+11.58; n=94	+10.26; n=86 / +12.92; n=88
		C	25.52; =89	+8.99; n=85	+8.11; n=77 / +8.48; n=83
		Average	26.67		
		Difference in change		T-C = +2.59 [+10%] NS	T-C = +2.15 [+8%] NS / T-C = +4.44 [+17%]**

In 'change' column: + improvement, - worsening of symptoms

In 'difference in change' cell: * statistically significant at p<0.05, ** statistically significant at p<0.01, NS not significant, NT not tested, + intervention of interest is more effective than comparator, - intervention of interest is less effective than comparator

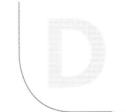

RCT	Measure		Baseline	Short term (<6 months)		Long term (≥6 months)
			Baseline	8 weeks	20 weeks	
Koumantakis 2005[49] T1 = Stabilisation-enhanced general exercise group T2 = general exercise group	Short-Form McGill Pain Questionnaire (responsive pain scale derived from the original McGill Pain Questionnaire)	T1	15.7(5.4); n=29	+6.1; n=29	+8.0; n=29	
		T2	16.3(6.4); n=26	+7.5; n=26	+6.1; n=26	
		Average	16			
		Difference in change		T1-T2 = -1.4 [-8.75% #] NS	T1-T2 = +1.9 [+11.9% #] NS	
	Pain VAS B (pain intensity over the past week on average)	T1	26.9(20.6); n=29	+14.6; n=29	+11.1; n=29	
		T2	40.2(24.6); n=26	+18.9; n=26	+22.4; n=26	
		Average	33.55			
		Difference in change		T1-T2 = -4.3 [-12.8% #] NS	T1-T2 = -11.3 [-33.7% #] NS	
	Pain VAS C (pain intensity over past month on average).	T1	49.9(26.4); n=29	+27.6; n=29	+26.8; n=29	
		T2	55.9(25.5); n=26	+28.1; n=26	+27.1; n=26	
		Average	52.9			
		Difference in change		T1-T2 = -0.5 [-0.95% #] NS	T1-T2 = -0.3 [-0.6% #] NS	

RCT	Measure		Baseline	Short term (<6 months)		Long term (≥6 months)
			Baseline	Post intervention		6 months
Manniche 1988(111)	0-10 pain score (10 = more pain)	T1	13.3 ;n=27	+7.6		+8.3
T1 = extension mobilising & strengthening (high intensity)		T2	14.0 ;n=29	+3.7		+2.9
T2 = extension mobilising & strengthening (low intensity)		T3	11.7 ;n=24	+2.5		+0.2
T3 = Physical mixed methods		Average	13			
		Difference in change		T1-T2 = +3.9 [+30%#] NT T1-T3 = +5.1 [+39%#] NT T2-T3 = +1.2 [+9%#] NT		T1-T2 = +5.4 [+42%#] NT T1-T3 = +8.1 [+62%#] NT T2-T3 = +2.7 [+21%#] NT
			Baseline	Post intervention	3 months	1 year
Manniche 1991(47)	Low Back Pain Rating Scale					
T1 = Intensive back strengthening group	N.B. only the difference in scoring is presented in the paper	T1	?; n=33	14.7	15.0	6.0
T2 = Modified back strengthening group		T2	?; n=36	5.7	7.0	6.0
C = alternative treatment†		C	?; n=36	2.0	5.5	0.0
		Average				
		Difference in change		T1-T2 = +9 * T1-C = +12.7 **	T1-T2 = +8.0 * T1-C = +9.5 *	T1-T2 = 0.0 NS T1-C = +6.0 NS

In 'change' column: + improvement, - worsening of symptoms

In 'difference in change' cell: * statistically significant at p<0.05, ** statistically significant at p<0.01, NS not significant, NT not tested, + intervention of interest is more effective than comparator, - intervention of interest is less effective than comparator

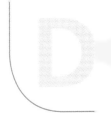

RCT	Measure	Baseline	Short term (<6 months)		Long term (≥6 months)
		Baseline	Post intervention	6 months	12 months
Mannion 1999 and 2001[56, 112] T1 = Physical mixed methods T2 = General exercises (with devices) T3 = General exercises (aerobic)	Average Pain Intensity 0-10 VAS				
		T1 4.4; n=46 T2 4.1; n=47 T3 4.2; n=44 Average 4.2	T1 +1.2; n=46 T2 +0.5; n=47 T3 +1.1; n=44	T1 +1.2; n=46 T2 +1.0; n=47 T3 +1.4; n=44	T1 +1.2; n=44 T2 +0.9; n=43 T3 +1.3; n=40
		Difference in change	T1-T2 = +0.7 [+17%#] NS T1-T3 = +0.1 [+2%#] NS T2-T3 = -0.6 [-14%#] NS	T1-T2 = +0.2 [+5%#] NS T1-T3 = -0.2 [-5%#] NS T2-T3 = -0.4 [-9%#] NS	T1-T2 = +0.3 [+7%#] NS T1-T3 = -0.1 [-2%#] NS T2-T3 = -0.4 [-9%#] NS
Martin 1986[46] T1 = flexion strengthening T2 = isometric strengthening C = placebo	Pain 0-5 scale (measured hourly) (data from graph)				
		T1 2.0; n=18 T2 1.8; n=19 C 2.3; n=12 Average (Total n=36) 2.0	T1 +0.3; n=12 T2 -0.2; n=12 C +0.9; n=12		
		Difference in change	T1-C = -0.6 [-30%#] NS T2-C = -1.1 [-55%#]* T1-T2 = +0.5 [+25%#] *		

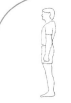

RCT	Measure		Baseline	Short term (<6 months)	Long term (≥6 months)
McIlveen 1998[72] T= Hydrotherapy C = Waitlist controls	Percentage of subjects who improved minimally 1 point on present pain intensity (a scale from 0-5)	T C Average	Baseline NA; n=45 NA; n=50 ?	Post intervention +33% +22% T-C = +11% NS	
Petersen 2002[48] T1= Intensive strengthening T2= McKenzie	Low back pain rating score 0-60	 T1 T2 Average Difference in change	Baseline 19; n=128 18.5; n=132 18.7	Post intervention +5; n=128 +8.5; n=132 T1-T2= -3 [-16%#] NS	2 months +2 ;n=128 +5.5 ; n=132 T1-T2= -3.5 [-19%#] NS	8 months +1; n=128 +4.5; n=132 T1-T2= -3.5 [-19%#] NS
Rasmussen-Barr 2003[71] T1 = ST group T2 = MT group	Pain VAS (10cm)	 T1 T2 Average Difference in change	Baseline 33; n=24 32; n=23 32.5	Post intervention +13; n=22 +8; n=19 T1-T2 = +5	3 months +19; n=17 +10; n=16 T1-T2 = +9 [+27.7%#] NS	12 months +20; n=17 +14; n=14 T1-T2 = +6 [+18.5%#] NS

In 'change' column: + improvement, - worsening of symptoms

In 'difference in change' cell: * statistically significant at p<0.05, ** statistically significant at p<0.01, NS not significant, NT not tested, + intervention of interest is more effective than comparator, - intervention of interest is less effective than comparator

RCT	Measure		Baseline	Short term (<6 months)	Long term (≥6 months)
Reilly 1989[69] T1 = supervised general exercises T2 = unsupervised general exercises	Pain 100mm VAS		Baseline	Post intervention	
		T1	81.2 ; n=20	+47.7 ; n=20	
		T2	82 ; n=20	+2.0 ; n=20	
		Average	81.6		
		Difference in change		T1-T2 = +45.7 [+56%#] NT	
Risch 1993[62] T = lumbar strengthening exercises C = wait list	West Haven Yale Multidimensional Pain Inventory, Pain subscale		Baseline	Post intervention	
		T	3.4 (1.6); n=31	+0.5 ; n=31	
		C	3.7 (1.6); n=23	-0.4 ; n=23	
		Average	3.6		
		Difference in change		T-C = +0.9 [+25%#] **	
Rittweger 2002[50] T1 = extension strengthening T2 = vibration exercises	Pain 0-10 VAS (endpoint data from graph)		Baseline	Post intervention	
		T1	4.5 n=30	+3.1 n=30	
		T2	4.2 n=30	+3.0 n=30	
		Average	4.35		
		Difference in change		T1-T2 = +0.1 [+2%#] NS	
Snook 1998[61] T1 = General exercises T2 = Control of early morning flexion	Pain intensity 0-10 point scale (10 = more pain)		Baseline		6 months
		T1	2.98; n=36		+0.19; n=36
		T2	2.14; n=24		+0.62; n=24
		Average	2.56		
		Difference in change			T1-T2 = -0.43 [-17%#] NT

RCT	Measure		Baseline	Short term (<6 months)	Long term (≥6 months)
Storheim 2003[54] T1 = Exercise regime T2 = cognitive intervention C = control group	Pain VAS: LBP (greatest pain at present) (0-100, 0=no pain)		Baseline	18 weeks	
		T1	53.2(23.2); n=30	+14.9; n=30	
		T2	55.7(19.6); n=34	+20.9; n=34	
		C	58.3(21.6); n=29	+10; n=29	
		Average	55.7		
		Difference in change		T1-T2 = -6 [-10.8% #] NS T1-C = +4.9 [+8.8% #] NS	
	Pain VAS: Lower Limb pain (greatest pain at present) (0-100, 0=no pain)		Baseline	18 weeks	
		T1	16.2(21.9); n=30	+2.1; n=30	
		T2	19.4(22.7); n=34	+5.8; n=34	
		C	28.8(29.3); n=29	+9.8; n=29	
		Average	21.5		
		Difference in change		T1-T2 = -3.7 [-17.2% #] NS T1-C = -7.7 [-35.8% #] NS	

In 'change' column: + improvement, - worsening of symptoms

In 'difference in change' cell: * statistically significant at p<0.05, ** statistically significant at p<0.01, NS not significant, NT not tested, + intervention of interest is more effective than comparator, - intervention of interest is less effective than comparator

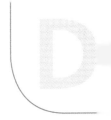

RCT	Measure		Baseline	Short term (<6 months)	Long term (≥6 months)
	Pain Diary Sensory (0-100, 0=no pain)		Baseline	18 weeks	
		T1	42.1(18.4); n=30	+11.3; n=30	
		T2	45.5(19.9); n=34	+9.6; n=34	
		C	43.0(19.6); n=29	+5.0; n=29	
		Average	43.5		
		Difference in change		T1-T2 = +1.7 [+3.91% #] NS T1-C = +6.3 [+14.5% #] NS	
	Pain Diary Affective (0-100, 0=no pain)		Baseline	18 weeks	
		T1	42.3(18.6); n=30	+10.4; n=30	
		T2	45.5(21.4); n=34	+9.7; n=34	
		C	43.7(21.6); n=29	+6.6; n=29	
		Average	43.8		
		Difference in change		T1-T2 = +0.7 [+1.6% #] NS T1-C = +3.8 [+8.7% #] NS	
Tritilanunt 2001[43] T = aerobic exercises C = flexion exercises	0-10 cm Vas score		Baseline	After 12 weeks of intervention	
		T	5.56; n=35	+3.26; n=35	
		C	5.42; n=33	+1.45; n=33	
		Average	5.49		
		Difference in change		T-C = +1.81** [+33% #]	

137

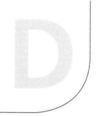

Table 3b: Main outcomes: Function

RCT	Measure		Baseline	Short term (<6 months)		Long term (≥6 months)
			Baseline	Post intervention	6 months	12 months
Turner, 1990[53] T1=Op-Behav T2=Op-Behav+ general exercise (quota-based) T3=General exercise (quota-based) C1=Wait list	McGill Pain Questionnaire	T1 T2 T3 C1 Average	20.96 n=25 25.54 n=24 19.42 n=24 21.17 n=23 21.77	+3.25 ;n=18 +10.75 ;n=18 +1.90 ;n=21 +0.22 ;n=19	+1.46 ;n=14 +12.25 ;n=14 +3.77 ;n=17	+4.55 ;n=17 +7.33 ;n=14 +4.48 ;n=16
		Difference in change		T1-T3 = +1.35 [+6%#] NS T2-T3 = +8.86 [+41%#] * T3-C1 = +1.68 [+8%#] NS	T1-T3 = -2.31 [-11%#] NS T2-T3 = +8.48 [+39%#] NS	T1- T3= +0.07 [+0%#] NS T2-T3= +2.85 [+13%#] NS

In 'change' column: + improvement, - worsening of symptoms

In 'difference in change' cell: * statistically significant at p<0.05, ** statistically significant at p<0.01, NS not significant, NT not tested, + intervention of interest is more effective than comparator, - intervention of interest is less effective than comparator

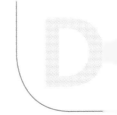

RCT	Measure		Baseline	Short term (<6 months)	Long term (≥6 months)
Torstensen 1998[55]	Pain intensity (back and leg) 200mm VAS		Baseline	Post intervention	12 months
T1 = general exercise		T1	78; n=71	+27.8; n=71	+32.7; n=71
T2 = physical mixed methods		T2	75.1; n=67	+28.8; n=67	+29.2; n=67
T3 = walking		T3	83.7; n=70	+2.2; n=70	+2.9; n=70
		Average	78.9		
		Difference in change		T1-T2 = +1.0 [+1%#] NS T1-T3 = +25.6 [+32%#] ** T2-T3 = +26.6 [+34#] **	T1-T2 = +3.5 [+4%#] NS T1-T3 = +29.8 [+38%#] ** T2-T3 = +26.3 [+33%#] **
UK BEAM 2004[63, 64]	Von Korff scale for pain (0-100) 0 is less pain		Baseline	3 months	12 months
T1= GP + exercise		T1	60.8 (17.6); n=310	+16.1 ;n=204	+19.3 ;n=200
T2= GP + manipulation		T2	61.5 ; n=353	+20.6 ;n=275	+19.8 ;n=264
T3= GP + exercise + manipulation		T3	60.0 ;n=333	+19.2 ;n=246	+20.3 ;n=245
C= GP		C	60.5 (17.6) ; n=338	+11.2; n=239	+13.1 ;n=235
		Average	60.7		
		Difference in change		T1-T2= -4.5 [7%#] NT T1-T3= -3.1 [-5%#] NT T1-C= +4.9 [+8%#] *	T1-T2= -0.5 [-0%#] NT T1-T3= -1 [-2%#] NT T1-C= +6.2 [+10%#] *
Yozbatiran 2004[68]	Pain VAS (10cm, 10 = worst pain)		Baseline	Post intervention	
T1 = fitness group		T1	5.06(2.28); n=15	+2.53; n=15	
T2 = aquafitness group		T2	5.46 (2.19); n=15	+3.53; n=15	
		Average	5.26		
		Difference in change		T1-T2 = -1 [-19.1%#] NT	

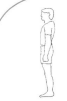

139

RCT	Measure		Baseline	Short term (<6 months)			Long term (≥6 months)	
Gur 2003[65] T1 = laser + exercise T2 = exercise T3 = laser	Roland Disability Questionnaire (0-24, high score = poor result)		Baseline	Post intervention				
		T1	17.8(4.6); n=25	+11.5; n=25				
		T2	15.1(4.2); n=25	+9.6; n=25				
		T3	16.3(3.9); n=25	+9.7; n=25				
		Average	16.4					
		Difference in change		T1-T2 = +1.9 [+11.6%#] NS T1-T3 = +1.8 [+10.98%#] NS				
	Modified Oswestry Disability Questionnaire (high score = poor result)		Baseline	Post intervention				
		T1	32.4(10.6); n=25	+17.6; n=25				
		T2	30.5(12.3); n=25	+16.9; n=25				
		T3	33.1(11.8); n=25	+16.4; n=25				
		Average	32					
		Difference in change		T1-T2 = +0.7 [+0.2%#] NS T1-T3 = +1.2 [+3.75%#] NS				

RCT	Measure		Baseline	1 month	2 months	3 months	6 months	9 months
Helmhout 2004[51] T1 = High intensity extension strengthening training T2 = Low intensity extension strengthening training	Roland Disability Questionnaire 24-item scale (0-24, 24 = high disability)		Baseline					
		T1	7.1(4.8); n=41	+2.6; n=41	+3.0; n=41	+2.9; n=39	+2.9; n=37	+3.9; n=33
		T2	7.9(4.8); n=40	+1.9; n=40	+2.2; n=40	+2.4; n=36	+3.6; n=33	+4.7; n=29
		Average	7.5					
		Difference in change		T1-T2 = +0.7 [+9.3% #] NS	T1-T2 = +0.8 [+10.7% #] NS	T1-T2 = +0.5 [+6.7% #] NS	T1-T2 = -0. [-9.3% #] NS	T1-T2 = -0.8 [-10.7% #] NS

In 'change' column: + improvement, - worsening of symptoms

In 'difference in change' cell: * statistically significant at p<0.05, ** statistically significant at p<0.01, NS not significant, NT not tested, + intervention of interest is more effective than comparator, - intervention of interest is less effective than comparator

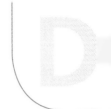

RCT	Measure		Baseline	Short term (<6 months)			Long term (≥6 months)	
	Oswestry Questionnaire: 10-item scale (0-100%, 100% = high rate of pain-indicated limitations).	T1	13.9(8.0); n=41	1 month: +0.7; n=41	2 months: +2.4; n=41	3 months: +3.1; n=39	6 months: +3.6; n=37	9 months: +4.9; n=33
		T2	17.4(13.2); n=40	+2.3; n=40	+4.2; n=40	+3.4; n=36	+3.8; n=33	+5.8; n=29
		Average	15.65					
		Difference in change		T1-T2 = -1.6 [-10.2%#] NS	T1-T2 = -1.8 [-11.5% #] NS	T1-T2 = -0.3 [-1.9%#] NS	T1-T2 = -0.2 [-1.3% #] NS	T1-T2 = -0.9 [-5.8% #] NS
Hemmila 1997[13] and 2002[14] T1 = (hom) exercise group (mobilising/strengthening) T2 = Bone-setting group T3 = physical mixed methods	Oswestry Disability Questionnaire	T1	19.4(9.5); n=35	6 weeks: +3.2; n=29	3 months: +2.9; n=35		6 months: +3.5; n=33	12 months: +2.2; n=32
		T2	23.7(11.6); n=44	+7.0; n=39	+5.1; n=43		+9.4; n=44	+8.4; n=44
		T3	18.1(7.7); n=34	+2.0; n=33	+4.0; n=33		+4.7; n=33	+4.4; n=32
		Average	20.4					
		Difference in change		T1-T2 = -3.8 [-18.6%#] NS; T1-T3 = +1.2 [+5.9%#] NS	T1-T2 = -2.2 [-10.8%#] NS; T1-T3 = -1.1 [-5.4%#] NS		T1-T2 = -5.9 [-28.9%#]*; T1-T3 = -1.2 [-5.9%#] NS	T1-T2 = -6.2 [-30.4%#]*; T1-T3 = -2.2 [-10.8%#] NS
Johannsen 1995[57] T1= general endurance exercise T2= general coordination exercises	Disability score 0-12 (12 questions on function, 1 point for impaired in function, 0 is no impairment)	T1	6; n=20	3 months: +4; n=13			6 months: +5; n=13	
		T2	5; n=20	+3; n=14			+3; n=14	
		Average	5.5					
		Difference in change		T1-T2= +1 [+18%#] NS			T1-T2= +2 [+46%#] NS	

RCT	Measure		Baseline	Short term (<6 months)	Long term (≥6 months)	
Jousset et al 2004[66] T1 = Functional restoration programme T2 = active individual physical therapy	French version of the Dallas Pain Questionnaire (0-100)^	ADL	Baseline		6 months	
			T1	53.7(16.7); n=42 0.3(16.7);		+17; n=42
			T2	n=41 52		+8.8; n=41
			Average			
			Difference in change			T1-T2 = +8.2 [+15.8% #] NT
		Work/ Leisure	Baseline		6 months	
			T1	54 (20.9); n=41		+20,n=42
			T2	58.7 (18.2); n=41 52		+17.4;n=41
			Average			
			Difference in change			T1-T2 = +2.6 [+4.6% #] NT
	Quebec Back Pain disability Scale (0-100)		Baseline		6 months	
			T1	34.6(15.4); n=42 31.6(15.9)		+12.6; n=42
			T2	;n=41 33.1		+8.7; n=41
			Average			
			Difference in change			T1-T2 = +3.9 [11.8% #] NT
Kankaanpaa 1999[67] T = General exercise (active rehab) C = Physical agents (passive rehab)	Pain & Disability Index		Baseline	Post intervention	6 months	12 months
			T	13.2 n=30	+2.4 n=30	+7.5 n=28	+7.5 n=27
			C	9.5 n=24	-1.4 n=24	-3.1 n=22	-1.9 n=22
			Average	11.4			
			Difference in change		T-C = +3.8 [+33%#] *	T-C = +10.6 [+93%#] **	T-C = +9.4 [+83%#] **

In 'change' column: + improvement, - worsening of symptoms

In 'difference in change' cell: * statistically significant at p<0.05, ** statistically significant at p<0.01, NS not significant, NT not tested, + intervention of interest is more effective than comparator, - intervention of interest is less effective than comparator

RCT	Measure		Baseline	Short term (<6 months)		Long term (≥6 months)	
Klaber Moffett 1999[58] T = exercise C = GP care	Roland Disability Questionnaire (0-24 points)		Baseline	6 weeks		6 months	12 months
		T	5.56 n=98	+2.86 n=94		+2.99 n=86	+3.19 n=88
		C	6.65 n=89	+1.94 n=85		+1.64 n=77	+1.77 n=83
		Average	6.11				
		Difference in change		T-C = +0.92 [+15%#] NS		T-C = +1.35 [+22%#] *	T-C = +1.42 [+23%#] *
Koumantakis[49] 2005 T1 = Stabilisation-enhanced general exercise group T2 = general exercise group	Roland-Morris disability Questionnaire (0-24, 0= no disability, 24 = highest disability)		Baseline	8 weeks		20 weeks	
		T1	9.2(4.6); n=29	+4.1; n=29		+4.7; n=29	
		T2	11.3(5.2); n=26	+6.6; n=26		+6.1; n=26	
		Average	10.25				
		Difference in change		T1-T2 = -2.5 [-24.4% #] *		T1-T2 = -1.4 [-13.7% #] NS	
Manniche 1991[111] T1 = Intensive back strengthening group T2 = Modified back strengthening group C = alternative treatment	Low Back Pain Rating Scale N.B. only the difference in scoring is presented in the paper		Baseline	Post intervention	3 months	1 year	
		T1	?; n=33	14.7	15.0	6.0	
		T2	?; n=36	5.7	7.0	6.0	
		C	?; n=36	2.0	5.5	0.0	
		Average	?				
		Difference in change		T1-T2 = +9 * **T1-C = +12.7 **	T1-T2 = +8.0 * T1-C = +9.5 *	T1-T2 = 0.0 NS T1-C = +6.0 NS	
Mannion 1999[56] and 2001[112] T1 = Physical mixed methods T2 = General exercise (with devices) T3 = General exercise (aerobic)	Roland Morris Disability Questionnaire		Baseline	6 weeks		6 months	12 months
		T1	7.9 n=46	+1.1 n=46		+0.2 n=46	+0.5n=44
		T2	7.7 n=47	+1.4 n=47		+2.3 n=47	+1.5n=43
		T3	8.0 n=44	+1.3 n=44		+2.3 n=44	+2.2n=40
		Average	7.87				
		Difference in change		T1 -T2 = -0.3 [-4%#] NS. T1-T3 = -0.2 [-3%#] NS. T2-T3 = +0.1 [+1%#] NS		T1 -T2 = -2.1 [-27%#] NS. T1-T3 = -2.1 [-27%#] NS. T2-T3 = 0 [0%#] NS	T1 -T2 = -1.0 [-13%#] NS. T1-T3 = -1.7 [-22%#] NS. T2-T3 = -0.7 [-9%#] NS

RCT	Measure	Baseline	Short term (<6 months)	Long term (≥6 months)
Martin 1986[46] T1 = flexion strengthening T2 = isometric strengthening C = placebo	Function 12 item questionnaire Read from graph	Baseline	Post intervention	
	T1	425 n=18	+175 n=12	
	T2	450 n=19	+50 n=12	
	C	390 n=12	-10 n=12	
	Average	426		
	Difference in change		T1-C = +185 [+44%#] NS T2-C = +60 [+14%#] NS T1-T2 = +125 [+30%#] NS	
McIlveen 1998[72] T= Hydrotherapy C = Waitlist controls	Percentage of subjects who improved minimally 10 points on Oswestry Disability Questionnaire	Baseline	Post intervention	
	T	NA; n=45	+27%	
	C	NA; n=50	+8%	
	Average	?		
			T-C = +19% *	
Petersen 2002[48] T1= Intensive strengthening T2= McKenzie	Disability score 0-100 (100 is more disabled)	Baseline	Post intervention / 2 months	8 months
	T1	39.3 ; n=128	+10.1; n=128 / +4.5; n=128	+6; n=128
	T2	36.7; n=132	+8.1; n=132 / +10; n=132	+5.9; n=132
	Average	38.0		
	Difference in change		T1-T2= +2 [+5%#] NS / T1-T2= -5.5 [-14%#] *	T1-T2= +0.1 [+0%#] NS

In 'change' column: + improvement, - worsening of symptoms

In 'difference in change' cell: * statistically significant at p<0.05, ** statistically significant at p<0.01, NS not significant, NT not tested, + intervention of interest is more effective than comparator, - intervention of interest is less effective than comparator

RCT	Measure		Baseline	Short term (<6 months)		Long term (≥6 months)
				Post intervention	3 months	12 months
Rasmussen-Barr 2003(71) T1 = ST group T2 = MT group	Oswestry Low Back-Pain Questionnaire	T1 T2 Average	18; n=24 14; n=23 16	+9; n=22 +2; n=19	+12; n=17 +1; n=16	+10; n=17 +6; n=14
		Difference in change		T1-T2 +7 43.75%# NS	T1-T2 = +11 [+68.75%#] NS	T1-T2 = +4 [+25%#] NS
	Disability Rating Index (measures perceived difficulty in performing 12 daily activities on VAS – 10cm, 0 = no difficulty)	T1 T2 Average	32; n=24 33; n=23 32.5	+10; n=22 +5; n=19	+20; n=17 +5; n=16	+19; n=17 +10; n=14
		Difference in change		T1-T2 +5 +15.4%# *	T1-T2 = +15 [+46.2%#] *	T1-T2 = +9 [+27.7%#] *
Risch 1993(62) T = extension strengthening C = wait list	SIP physical dysfunction	T C Average	9.1 n=31 15.2 n=23 12.2	+1.4 n=31 -4.1 n=23		
		Difference in change		T-C = +5.5 [+45%#] *		

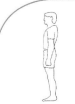

RCT	Measure		Baseline	Short term (<6 months)	Long term (≥6 months)
Rittweger 2002[50]	Pain Disability Index		Baseline	Post intervention	6 months
T1 = extension strengthening		T1	20.3 n=30	+9.8 n=?	+8.3 n=?
T2 = vibration exercises		T2	20.7 n=30	+9.1 n=?	+5.9 n=?
		Average	20.5		
		Difference in change		T1-T2 = +0.7 [+3%#] NS	T1-T2 = +2.4 [+12%#] NS
Shaughnessy 2004[70]	Roland-Morris disability Questionnaire (high score = high disability)		Baseline	10 weeks	
T1 = Lumbar stabilisation programme		T1	10(4.1); n=20	+4.9; n=20	
C = no intervention		C	10.7(5.6); n=21	-0.6; n=21	
		Average	10.35		
		Difference in change		T1-C = +5.5 [53.1% #] **	
	Oswestry Disability Questionnaire (high score = high disability)		Baseline	10 weeks	
		T1	37(13); n=20	+11; n=20	
		C	41(15); n=21	-3; n=21	
		Average	39		
		Difference in change		T1-C = +14 [+35.9% #] **	
Storheim 2003[54]	Roland Morris questionnaire (0-24, 0=best score)		Baseline	18 weeks	
T1 = Exercise regime		T1	8.2(3.5); n=30	+2.1; n=30	
T2 = cognitive intervention		T2	8.9(3.4); n=34	+3.5; n=34	
C = control group		C	9.3(3.6); n=29	+1.6; n=29	
		Average	8.8		
		Difference in change		T1-T2 = -1.4 [-15.9% #] NS	
				T1-C = +0.5 [+5.7% #] NS	

In 'change' column: + improvement, - worsening of symptoms

In 'difference in change' cell: * statistically significant at p<0.05, ** statistically significant at p<0.01, NS not significant, NT not tested, + intervention of interest is more effective than comparator, - intervention of interest is less effective than comparator

RCT	Measure		Baseline	Short term (<6 months)	Long term (≥6 months)
			Baseline	Post intervention	12 months
Torstensen 1998[55] T1 = general exercise T2 = physical mixed methods T3 = walking	Oswestry Low Back Pain Disability Questionnaire	T1	51.7 n=71	+5.5 n=71	+7.6 n=71
		T2	49.4 n=67	+2.5 n=67	+6.4 n=67
		T3	50.0 n=70	-2.7 n=70	-0.6 n=70
		Average	50.4		
		Difference in change		T1-T2 = +2.5 [+5%#] NS T1-T3 = +8.2 [+16%#] ** T2-T3 = +5.2 [+10%#] **	T1-T2 = +1.2 [+2%#] NS T1-T3 = +8.2 [+16%#] ** T2-T3 = +7.0 [+14%#] **
			Baseline	Post intervention	6 months / 12 months
Turner, 1990[53] T1=Op-Behav T2=Op-Behav+ general exercise (quota-based) T3=General exercise (quota-based) C=Wait list	Sickness Impact Profile	T1	7.90 n=25	+3.18 n=18	6 months: +0.30 n=14 / 12 months: +2.65 n=17
		T2	8.50 n=24	+4.87 n=18	+3.99 n=14 / +3.75 n=14
		T3	8.42 n=24	+2.93 n=21	+2.17 n=17 / +3.69 n=16
		C	6.24 n=23	+0.87 n=19	- / -
		Average	7.77		
		Difference in change		T1-T3 = +0.25 [+3%#] NS T2-T3 = +1.94 [+25%#] * T3-C1 = 2.06 [27%#] NS	6 months: T1-T3=-1.87 [-24%#] NS T2-T3= +1.82 [+23%#] NS 12 months: T1-T3=-1.04 [-13%#] NS T2-T3= +0.06 [+0%#] NS

RCT	Measure		Baseline	Short term (<6 months)	Long term (≥6 months)
UK BEAM 2004[63, 64] T1= GP + exercise T2= GP + manipulation T3= GP + exercise + manipulation C = GP	Roland Disability Questionnaire (0-24) 0 = best		Baseline	3 months	12 months
		T1	9.2 (4.3) ;n=310	+3.7; n=225	+3.5 ; n=248
		T2	8.9 ; n=353	+3.8; n=273	+3.8; n=273
		T3	9.0 ;n=333	+4.2; n=258	+4.3; n=257
		C	9.0 (3.9); n=338	+2.3 ; n=256	+2.9; n=248
		Average	9.0		
		Difference in change		T1-T2= -0.1 [-1%#] NT T1-T3= -0.5 [-6%#] NT T1-C= +1.4 [+16%#] *	T1-T2= -0.3 [-3%#] NT T1-T3= -0.8 [-9%#] NT T1-C= +0.6 [+7%#] NS
	Modified Von Korff Scale for disability (0-100) 0=best		Baseline	3 months	12 months
		T1	47.7 (22.6); n=310	+18.0; n=205	+18.0; n=202
		T2	46.8 ;n=353	+15.7; n=275	+17.0; n=262
		T3	45.0 ;n=333	+16.0; n=246	+16.9; n=246
		C	44.9 (21.0); n=338	+10.1; n=239	+10.4; n=235
		Average	46.1		
		Difference in change		T1-T2= +2.3 [+5%#] NT T1-T3= +2 [+4%#] NT T1-C= +7.9 [+17%#] *	T1-T2= +1 [+2%#] NT T1-T3= +1.1 [+2%#] NT T1-C= +7.6 [+16%#] NS
Yozbatiran 2004[68] T1 = fitness group T2 = aquafitness group	Oswestry low back disability questionnaire (high score = high disability)		Baseline	Post intervention	
		T1	38.4 (14.32);n=15	+17.34; n=15	
		T2	40 (20.14); n=15	+19.34; n=15	
		Average	39.2		
		Difference in change		T1-T2 = -2 [-5.1%#] NT	

In 'change' column: + improvement, - worsening of symptoms

In 'difference in change' cell: * statistically significant at p<0.05, ** statistically significant at p<0.01, NS not significant, NT not tested, + intervention of interest is more effective than comparator, - intervention of interest is less effective than comparator

Table 3c: Main outcomes: Psychological status

RCT	Measure		Baseline	Short term (<6 months)			Long term (≥6 months)	
				1 month	2 months	3 months	6 months	9 months
Helmhout 2004[51] T1 = High intensity extension strengthening Training T2 = Low intensity extension strengthening training	Tampa scale for kinesiophobia (TSK) (17-item scale, 4-68 points, high score indicates high degree of fear of movement).	T1	37.0(6.1); n=41	+0.5; n=41	+0.5; n=41	+2.0; n=39	+2.0; n=37	+2.1; n=33
		T2	40.0(7.0); n=40	+1.2; n=40	+3.1; n=40	+2.9; n=36	+3.5; n=33	+6.2; n=29
		Average	38.5					
		Difference in change		T1-T2 = -0.7 [-1.8% #] NS	T1-T2 = -2.6 [-6.8% #] *	T1-T2 = -0.9 [-2.3% #] NS	T1-T2 = -1.5 [-3.9% #] NS	T1-T2 = -4.1 [-10.6% #] *
Jousset et al 2004[66] T1 = Functional restoration programme T2 = active individual physical therapy	French version of the Dallas Pain Questionnaire (0-100)^	T1	40.6(25.3); n=41				+19; n=42	
		T2	31.8(23.1); n=41				+4; n=41	
		Average	36.2					
		Difference in change					T1-T2 = +15 [+41.4% #] NT	
	Psychological profile: Hospital Anxiety Depression Scale (HAD)	T1	17(6.5); n=42				+4.3; n=42	
		T2	14.3(6.1); n=41				+0.9; n=41	
		Average	15.65					
		Difference in change					T1-T2 = +3.4 [21.8% #] NT	

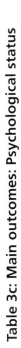
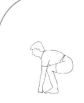

RCT	Measure		Baseline	Short term (<6 months)		Long term (≥6 months)
				8 weeks	20 weeks	
Koumantakis 2005[49] T1 = Stabilisation-enhanced general exercise group T2 = general exercise group	Tampa Scale of Kinesiophobia (Fear of movement/re-injury) (17 item scale, scores range from 17=no fear to 68 = highest fear)	T1	37.6(6.3); n=29	+3.9; n=29	+6.1; n=29	
		T2	40.5(8.9); n=26	**+5.4; n=26**	+7.6; n=26	
		Average	39.05			
		Difference in change	20 weeks	**T1-T2 = -1.5 [-3.8% #] NS**	T1-T2 = -1.5 [-3.8% #] NS	
	Pain Self-Efficacy Questionnaire (10-item scale, scores 0= no self-efficacy, 60 = highest self efficacy).	T1	42.0(12.3); n=29	+7.2; n=29	+9.2; n=29	
		T2	37.3(11.1); n=26	+10.8; n=26	+11.6; n=26	
		Average	39.65			
		Difference in change		T1-T2 = -3.6 [-9.1% #] NS	T1-T2 = -2.4 [-6.1% #] NS	
	Pain Locus of Control Scale 1. Pain Control	T1	12.4(4.5); n=29	0; n=29	-1.5; n=29	
		T2	11.2(6.0); n=26	+0.1; n=26	-1.3; n=26	
		Average	11.8			
		Difference in change		T1-T2 = -0.1 [-0.85% #] NS	T1-T2 = -0.2 [-1.69% #] NS	
	2. Pain Responsibility	T1	8.0(1.9); n=29	+1.4; n=29	+1.7; n=29	
		T2	8.0(2.4); n=26	+1.3; n=26	+2.2; n=26	
		Average	8.0			
		Difference in change		T1-T2 = +0.1 [+1.25% #] NS	T1-T2 = -0.5 [-6.25% #] NS	

In 'change' column: + improvement, - worsening of symptoms

In 'difference in change' cell: * statistically significant at p<0.05, ** statistically significant at p<0.01, NS not significant, NT not tested, + intervention of interest is more effective than comparator, - intervention of interest is less effective than comparator

RCT	Measure		Baseline	Short term (<6 months)	Long term (≥6 months)
Mannion 1999[56, 112] and 2001[112] T1 = Physical mixed methods T2 = General exercise (devices) T3 = General exercise (aerobic)	Modified Zung questionnaire (score 0-60)			Post intervention	6 months
		T1	13.5 n=46	-0.2 n=46	-1.7 n=46
		T2	12.1 n=47	+0.9 n=47	+0.7 n=47
		T3	14.9 n=44	+2.6 n=44	+1.9 n=44
		Average	13.5		
		Difference in change		T1-T2 = -1.1 [-8%#] NS T1-T3 = -2.8 [-21%#] NS T2-T3 = -1.7 [-13%#] NS	T1-T2 = -2.4 [-18%#] * T1-T3 = -3.6 [-27%#] * T2-T3 = -1.2 [-9%#] NS
Rittweger 2002[50] T1 = extension strengthening T2 = vibration exercises	Allgemeine Depression Skala (normals in range 40-60)			Post intervention	6 months
		T1	48.0 n=30	+4.3 n=?	+4.3 n=?
		T2	45.5 n=30	+2.5 n=?	-1.0 n=?
		Average	46.8		
		Difference in change		T1-T2 = +1.8 [+4%#] NT	T1-T2 = +5.3 [+11%#] NT
Storheim 2003[54] T1 = Exercise regime T2 = cognitive intervention C = control group	Fear-Avoidance Belief Questionnaire (FABQ) Split into 2 categories: physical activity, work. The 2 are added together here.		Baseline	18 weeks	
		T1	39.2; n=30	+7.1; n=30	
		T2	40.8; n=34	+9; n=34	
		C	43.7; n=29	-0.2; n=29	
		Average	41.2		
		Difference in change		T1-T2 = -1.9 [-4.6% #] NS T1-C = +7.3 [+17.7% #] *	
	Hopkins Symptom Checklist (HSCL-25) for emotional distress.		Baseline	18 weeks	
		T1	1.4(0.4); n=30	+0.006; n=30	
		T2	1.5(0.4); n=34	+0.2; n=34	
		C	1.6(0.4); n=29	-0.003; n=29	
		Average	1.5		
		Difference in change		T1-T2 = -0.19 [-12.9% #] * T1-C = +0.009 [+0.6 #] NS	

RCT	Measure		Baseline	Short term (<6 months)	Long term (≥6 months)
	Fear avoidance beliefs questionnaire 0-24 (0=best)		Baseline	3 months	12 months
UK BEAM 2004[63, 64]		T1	15.0 (5.3) ; n=310	+4.2 ;n=200	+3.4 ;n=187
T1= GP + exercise		T2	14.9 ; n=353	+3.0 ;n=271	+2.0 ;n=260
T2= GP + manipulation		T3	15.0 ; n=333	+4.3 ;n=245	+3.4 ;n=204
T3= GP + exercise + manipulation		C	14.9 (5.1) ; n=338	+1.8 ;n=236	+2.1 ;n=208
C= GP		Ave	15.0		
		Difference in change		T1-T2=+1.2 [+8%#] NT T1-T3= -0.1 [0%#] NT T1-C= +2.4 [+16%#] *	T1-T2= +1.4 [+9%#] NT T1-T3= 0 [0%#] NT T1-C= +1.3 [+9%#] NS

In 'change' column: + improvement, - worsening of symptoms

In 'difference in change' cell: * statistically significant at $p<0.05$, ** statistically significant at $p<0.01$, NS not significant, NT not tested, + intervention of interest is more effective than comparator, - intervention of interest is less effective than comparator

Table 3d: Main outcomes: sick leave/return to work

RCT	Measure		Baseline	Short term (<6 months)		Long term (≥6 months)
Hemmila 2002[13, 14]	Sick-leave days for back pain		Year before treatment			Year after treatment
T1 = Exercise group		T1	2.5(5.9) ;n=35			-1 ;n=32
T2 = Bone-setting group		T2	8.7(28) ;n=45			+0.8 ;n=44
T3 = physiotherapy		T3	3.2(11); n=34			+2 ;n=32
		Average	14.4			
		Difference in change				T1-T2 = -1.8 [-12.5%#] NS T1-T3 = -3 [-20.8%#] NS
Jousset et al 2004[66]	No of sick-leave days (mean)		Baseline			6 months
T1 = Functional restoration programme		T1	?;n=42			28.7(44.6);n=42
T2 = active individual physical therapy		T2	?;n=41			48.3(66);n=41
		Average	?			
		Difference in change				T1-T2 = 19.4 NS
Petersen 2002[48]	Number of patients on sick leave		Baseline	Post intervention	2 months	8 months
T1= Intensive strengthening		T1	26 out of 86 (30%)	22 out of 86 (26%)	12 out of 86 (14%)	7 out of 86 (8%)
T2= McKenzie		T2	29 out of 94 (31%)	14 out of 94 (15%)	9 out of 94 (10%)	7 out of 94 (7%)
		Average	?			
		Difference		T1-T2= 11% NS	T1-T2= 4% NS	T1-T2= 1% NS

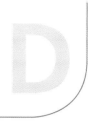

Table 3e Main Outcome: Costs

RCT	Measure		Baseline	Short term (<6 months)	Long term (≥6 months)
Klaber Moffett 1999[58] T = General exercise C = GP care	Mean health care costs per patient	T		£86.83 (105.19)	
		C		£111.05 (205.11)	
		Difference		£24.23ns (95%CI: -29.94, 78.89)	
	Mean total costs per patient	T		£360.15 (582.27)	
		C		£508.43 (1108.79)	
		Difference		£148.28ns (95%CI: -145.92, 442.48)	
Mannion 1999[56] and 2001[112] T1 = General exercise (aerobics) T2 = General exercise (with devices) T3 = Mixed methods physical	Mean health care costs per patient	T1		288 SFr	
		T2		1120 SFr	
		T3		960 SFr	
		Difference		T1-T2 = -832 SFr T1-T3 = -672 SFr T2-T3 = 160 SFr	

NOK = Norwegian Kroner; SFr = Swiss Francs

*p<0.05; **p<0.01; ***p<0.001; ns = not significant; CC = Cannot calculate difference between groups

In 'change' column: + improvement, - worsening of symptoms

In 'difference in change' cell: * statistically significant at p<0.05, ** statistically significant at p<0.01, NS not significant, NT not tested, + intervention of interest is more effective than comparator, - intervention of interest is less effective than comparator

154

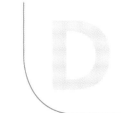

RCT	Measure		Baseline	Short term (<6 months)	Long term (≥6 months)
Torstensen 1998[55] T1 = General exercise T2 = Physical mixed methods T3 = Walking	Direct costs of treatments	T1 T2 T3		77 NOK x 36 sessions = 2772 NOK 120 NOK x 36 sessions = 4320 NOK 0 NOK	
		Difference		T1-T2 = -1548 NOK T1-T3 = 2772 NOK T2-T3 = 4320 NOK	
	Direct costs of sick leave over 15 months	T1 T2 T3		11,757 days x 600 NOK = 7,054,200 NOK 9967 days x 600 NOK = 5,980,200 NOK 13,587 days x 600 NOK = 8,152,200 NOK	
		Difference		T1-T2 = 1,074,000 NOK T1-T3 = -1,098,000 NOK T2-T3 = -2,172,000 NOK	
UK BEAM 2004[63, 64] T1= GP + exercise T2= GP + manipulation T3= GP + exercise + manipulation C = GP	Reported mean costs (SD) of health care over 12 months	T1 T2 T3 C		£486 (907) £541 (768) £471 (490) £346 (602)	
		Difference		T1-T2 = +55 T1-T3=-15 T1-C=-140	

In 'change' column: + improvement, - worsening of symptoms

In 'difference in change' cell: * statistically significant at p<0.05, ** statistically significant at p<0.01, NS not significant, NT not tested, + intervention of interest is more effective than comparator, - intervention of interest is less effective than comparator

Table 4: Excluded Systematic Reviews and Randomised Controlled Trials

SR	Reason for exclusion
Clare et al 2004[115]	Trials identified by the paper all involved acute low back pain with no separation of results if the patient had had pain for longer.
Colle 2002[116]	Examined impact of quality scales on systematic review's conclusions
Dagfinrud et al 2005[117]	General physiotherapy for ankylosing spondylitis – not just low back pain aspect of it.
Faas 1996[118]	Last search in 1995, only 7 eligible trials identified
Hilde 1998[119]	Last search 1995, only 6 eligible trials identified
Kool et al 2004[120] (Meta-analysis)	Looked at patients with pain longer then 4/52.
Mior 2001[121]	Re-examines Van Tulder systematic review[122]
Rainville et al 2004[123]	Non-systematic review
Smidt 2005[124]	Summary of systematic reviews
Van Tulder 2000[125]	Last search 1999, only 15 eligible trials identified
RCT	**Reason for exclusion**
Analay et al 2003[126]	Ankylosing Spondylitis patients, length of time of LBP not identified.
Aure 2003[127]	Combination of therapies
Bentsen 1997[128]	Includes patients with less than 6 weeks of LBP
Bronfort 2000[129]	LBP 2-12 weeks, the results were not segregated according to duration
Brox 2003[130]	Combination of therapies
Cherkin 1998[131]	LBP >7 days, the results were not segregated according to duration
Chok 1999[132]	LBP >7 days – 7 weeks, the results were not segregated according to duration
Coxhead 1981[133]	LBP any duration, results not segregated according to duration
Davies 1979[134]	LBP any duration, results not segregated according to duration
Descarreaux 2002[135]	LBP >7 days, the results were not segregated according to duration
Deyo 1990[77]	Used exercise in combination with TENS or sham TENS
Fernandez-de-las-Penas 2005[136]	Only looked at patients with ankylosing spondylitis, didn't different lumbar spine nor length of time with pain in the results.

In 'change' column: + improvement, - worsening of symptoms

In 'difference in change' cell: * statistically significant at $p<0.05$, ** statistically significant at $p<0.01$, NS not significant, NT not tested, + intervention of interest is more effective than comparator, - intervention of interest is less effective than comparator

RCT	Reason for exclusion
Frost 1995[137]	Combination of therapies
Frost 1998[78]	Combination of therapies
Ghoname 1999[138]	Cross over design
Glaser 2001[139]	Combination of therapies
Grunnesjo et al 2004[140]	Didn't separate results for A and SA patients.
Hagen 2003[141]	Used exercise in combination with other interventions
Hagins 1999[142]	Healthy participants
Hansen 1993[143]	Population studied included patients with LBP of less than 4 weeks duration, with no segregation of results according to duration.
Holmes 1996[144]	Pain free control group
Keller et al 2003[145]	Outcome measures not relevant (muscle strength, cross-sectional area and density) – follow up study to the Brox et al fusion vs exs study.
Klaber Moffett 1986[103]	Used a combination of interventions
Klaber Moffett 2004[146]	Sub-analysis of Klaber Moffett 1999, which included SA LBP
Klein 1990[79]	Combination of therapies
Langridge 1988[147]	Uncontrolled prospective study
LeFort 1994[148]	Uncontrolled prospective study
Lewis 2005[149]	Used manual therapy in combination with exercise
Lidstrom 1970[80]	Combination of intervention
Lindstrom 1992[74] (Physical Therapy)	Combination of interventions
Lindstrom 1992[75] (Spine paper)	Same paper as the other Lindstrom 1992 (Physical Therapy) but irrelevant outcomes to this investigation.
Ljunggren 1997[150]	LBP any duration, results not segregated according to duration
Long et al 2004[151]	Looked at patients with A, SA and C LBP but didn't separate the results.
Manniche 1993[152]	Ex-surgery patients
Niemisto 2003[153]	Combined therapies

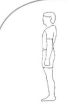

RCT	Reason for exclusion
O'Sullivan 1997[154]	Patients had radiologically confirmed diagnosis of spondylosis or spondylothesis
O'Sullivan 1998[155]	Irrelevant outcome measures. (electromyography).
Risch 1993[62]	LBP any duration, results not segregated according to duration
Rittweger 2002[50]	Already covered in previous table (evidence tables exercise old – the original tables)
Roberts 1995[156]	Retrospective audit
Sachs 1994[157]	Patients allocated into two groups by birth date, not a truly random procedure
Sjogren 1997[158]	Patients allocated into two groups by alternate allocation, not a truly random procedure.
Soukup 1999[159]	Prevention study
Staal et al 2004[160]	Only 4/52 duration of pain
Sweetman 1993[161]	LBP any duration, results not segregated according to duration
Timm 1994[162]	LBP after laminectomy
Verna 2002[163]	Healthy participants
Yelland 2003[164]	Non UK physiotherapy interventions
Zybergold 1981[165]	LBP any duration, results not segregated according to duration

In 'change' column: + improvement, - worsening of symptoms

In 'difference in change' cell: * statistically significant at p<0.05, ** statistically significant at p<0.01, NS not significant, NT not tested, + intervention of interest is more effective than comparator, - intervention of interest is less effective than comparator

Appendix E1

Exercise for people with persistent low back pain (LBP)

First round: before discussion

Please click to mark **one box only** for each question below.

Take into account **all your knowledge** and **experience** (clinical, research, service user) and the **evidence review** (attached) when answering these questions.

Refer also to the definitions of the exercises in the evidence review.

Statement	Agree	Neither agree nor disagree	Disagree
Reducing pain for people with persistent LBP			
Mobilising exercises are more effective than no active intervention in reducing pain	☐	☐	☐
Unsupervised walking is more effective than no active intervention in reducing pain	☐	☐	☐
Core stability exercises are more effective than no active intervention in reducing pain	☐	☐	☐
Hydrotherapy exercises are more effective than no active intervention in reducing pain	☐	☐	☐
Improving function for people with persistent LBP			
Mobilising exercises are more effective than no active intervention in improving function	☐	☐	☐
Strengthening exercises are more effective than no active intervention in improving function	☐	☐	☐
Unsupervised walking is more effective than no active intervention in improving function	☐	☐	☐
Core stability exercises are more effective than no active intervention in improving function	☐	☐	☐
Hydrotherapy exercises are more effective than no active intervention in improving function	☐	☐	☐
McKenzie exercises are more effective than no active intervention in improving function	☐	☐	☐
Improving psychological status for people with persistent LBP			
Mobilising exercises are more effective than no active intervention in improving psychological status	☐	☐	☐
Strengthening exercises are more effective than no active intervention in improving psychological status	☐	☐	☐
Unsupervised walking is more effective than no active intervention in improving psychological status	☐	☐	☐

Statement	Agree	Neither agree nor disagree	Disagree
Organised aerobic exercises are more effective than no active intervention in improving psychological status	☐	☐	☐
Combined exercises are more effective than no active intervention in improving psychological status	☐	☐	☐
Core stability exercises are more effective than no active intervention in improving psychological status	☐	☐	☐
Hydrotherapy exercises are more effective than no active intervention in improving psychological status	☐	☐	☐
McKenzie exercises are more effective than no active intervention in improving psychological status	☐	☐	☐

Either email completed form, by **Friday 2nd December 2005**, to Susan Williams at: williamss@csp.org.uk or return hard copy to:

Susan Williams, Administrator (R & CE Unit),
The Chartered Society of Physiotherapy,
14 Bedford Row, London WC1R 4ED.

The next stages in reaching consensus

- Where the group are not agreed, statements will be discussed on the iCSP back pain guidelines site from 8th December. Please join this debate.

- After the debate you will be asked to complete another, similar, questionnaire in the first week of January. The second round questionnaire will include an indication of how the group voted in the first round.

Thank your help in producing these guidelines!

Note to readers

The question:

Hydrotherapy exercises are more effective than no active intervention in improving function was included in this questionnaire but there is research evidence for this (section 4.8). The reason is that the research evidence was added to the systematic review after this questionnaire was sent out. The research evidence took precedence over the nominal group consensus evidence hence the latter was discarded.

Appendix E2

The iCSP discussion

This gives a flavour of the iCSP discussion which took place between completion of the first and second round consensus questionnaires. These questions were discussed because research evidence does not answer them. The nominal consensus group were asked to share their personal opinions, experience and unpublished workplace audits and thus much is unreferenced.

Key to abbreviations used in this appendix

ROM – range of motion
L/S – lumbar spine
Th/S
↓ – decreased / decreasing / decreases
↑ – increased / increasing / increases

Reducing pain for people with persistent LBP	
Consensus question with 1st round agreement	Some discussion points
1. Mobilising exercises are more effective than no active intervention in reducing pain agree mid disagree 60% 24% 16%	**For** Indicated where ROM is ↓ in Th/S, L/S and hips ↓ ROM in the L/S may be a risk factor for ↓ LBP[166] A subgroup of people with persistent LBP have limited hip ROM[167] Mobilising exercise must be better than no intervention May be useful where ROM is ↓ at the end of range Done daily they are beneficial in ↓ pain People return to clinic for review of mobilising exercises given years ago, they stop exercising when their pain ↓ Useful stepping stone to active rehabilitation Where there are psychosocial issues mobilising exercises should be active rather than therapist assisted **Against / mid** It is better to focus on ↑ function rather than on ↓ pain Often ↓ ROM likely to be short lived in LBP Difficult to believe that pain will be ↓ long-term

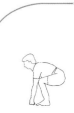

Reducing pain for people with persistent LBP	
2. Unsupervised walking is more effective than no active intervention in reducing pain agree 56% mid 24% disagree 20%	**For** Walking is useful Perhaps walking is shown to be less effective than general exercises or physical mixed methods[55] because the latter were more controlled and physiotherapists gave individuals more attention Activity is better than no activity Participation may be an issue so a good assessment of people's beliefs and willingness to participate is necessary Long-term compliance may be good **Against / mid** Things are too complex to be summarised by such a simple statement Walking may or may not ↓ pain
3. Core stability exercises are more effective than no active intervention in reducing pain agree 56% mid 24% disagree 20%	**For** Trials soon to be published found that core stabilising exercises ↓ pain effectively (although the comparison was not no treatment) Any intervention is likely to be better than no active intervention They are effective but training should be done in functional position Ideal for acute LBP but there is no evidence of their effectiveness for persistent LBP A workplace audit has suggested that combined aerobic and core stability exercises may be effective **Against / mid** For a more active person this kind of exercise may seem too minimal to be effective This works for a select subgroup of people and should not be used indiscriminately They may or may not improve muscle control
4. Hydrotherapy exercises are more effective than no active intervention in reducing pain agree 52% mid 32% disagree 16%	**For** BackCare self-help groups notice ↑ pain when they miss sessions / a qualitative student study supports this Where fear is a factor then exercising in the warm water will feel safer, ↓ pain and may be preferred by people with persistent LBP Excellent where co-morbidity makes dry land exercise difficult Compliance may be better for those choosing hydrotherapy as a way of exercising All types of exercise can be included in a hydrotherapy programme A workplace questionnaire of 110 people with persistent LBP found 62% reported ↓ pain after a course of hydrotherapy Any form of exercise is beneficial, hydrotherapy must be recommended Immersion has a physiological effect on nerve conduction that ↓ pain Exercise in water may be chosen by people with persistent LBP as a way to continue exercising People who benefit from hydrotherapy are often extremely enthusiastic making it difficult to separate pain ↓ from overall outcome **Against / mid** May not be transference to dry land

Reducing pain for people with persistent LBP	
	↓ pain in the short-term may increase dependency and fear of normal activity long-term
	But as long as people are not over medicalised self-referral / self-help groups demonstrates the patient is in control and it is unimportant if there are no measurable effects on dry land
Improving function for people with persistent LBP	
5. Mobilising exercises are more effective than no active intervention in improving function agree mid disagree 64% 28% 8%	**For** Mobilising exercises may ↑ ROM but do not necessarily ↑ function e.g., walking, work, lifting Can help a person feel ↑ confidence in getting on with normal activities and should therefore lead to ↑ function It is right that clinicians often rate mobilising exercises highly for those who are immobile or have ↓ ROM late in their rehabilitation It seems reasonable to expect some benefit from movement, the mechanism by which this happens is likely to be complex involving factors such as ↓ fear of movement
6. Strengthening exercises are more effective than no active intervention in improving function agree mid disagree 80% 8% 12%	No discussion, consensus reached in the first round questionnaire

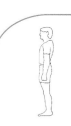

Reducing pain for people with persistent LBP	
7. Unsupervised walking is more effective than no active intervention in improving function agree mid disagree 76% 24% 0%	Consensus was reached in the first round questionnaire but at the time of setting up the conference, before the final results had been collated, only 74% consensus was achieved. This discussion has been included because important points were made. **For** If a person is willing and able to walk it is surely more effective than doing nothing In the longer term people are more likely to adhere to an unsupervised programme than have to attend a session on a particular time and date[168] Walking has to be better than sitting in front of the TV all day! A few may not comply due to fear avoidance but for the vast majority walking is likely to be effective Current guidelines recommend activity and include walking Walking is a practical and feasible means to staying active and being fit which is the key to managing LBP **Against / mid** Psychosocial factors may adversely affect compliance with this, it shouldn't be recommended as a form of treatment Many walk as much as they are able already Some advised to walk appear to fatigue and end up with muscle pain around the hips, thighs and L/S Advice on pacing is essential Reassessment is necessary if no benefit is experienced Compliance may be an issue
8. Core stability exercises are more effective than no active intervention in improving function agree mid disagree 72% 16% 12%	**For** A soon to be published paper found equal benefits for a spinal stability approach and 'standard physiotherapy' with advice to be active Any study comparing core stability exercises, delivered by physiotherapists, with no active intervention, will demonstrate improved function using a robust tool **Against / mid** Stability exercises may or may not improve function

Reducing pain for people with persistent LBP	
9. Hydrotherapy exercises are more effective than no active intervention in improving function agree mid disagree 64% 28% 8%	This question went to consensus because the Ib evidence that hydrotherapy is more effective than a waiting list control group in improving function (short-term)[72] had not been added to the evidence review at the time of distributing the questionnaire. **For** A workplace questionnaire of 110 people with persistent LBP found 51% reported that they were 'more able to do what they wanted to do' after a course of hydrotherapy
10. McKenzie exercises are more effective than no active intervention in improving function agree mid disagree 60% 24% 16%	**For** Petersen[48] found McKenzie exercises at least as effective as strengthening exercises for ↓ pain, ↑ function and ↑ return to work. Donchin[45] found strengthening exercises ↓ pain. Extrapolating from these McKenzie exercises should improve function. It is impossible to conclude that McKenzie exercises are not better than 'no active intervention' in ↑ function A systematic review (5 trials) of McKenzie exercises for spinal pain concluded that McKenzie therapy results in a greater ↓ in pain and ↑ function (short-term) than standard therapies.[115] The most appropriate answer is agree. The European guidelines group concluded that no specific form of exercise has been clearly found to be better than another so it is likely that McKenzie exercise is more effective than no treatment. It is surprising that anybody might disagree and the same applies to any other forms of exercise under discussion?
Improving psychological status for people with persistent LBP	
11. Mobilising exercises are more effective than no active intervention in improving psychological status agree mid disagree 56% 32% 12%	**For** If mobilising exercises can ↓ pain and ↑ function why would anybody think that they do not also ↑ psychological status more effectively than no active intervention. Physiotherapists tend to target ↓ pain and ↑ function but pain related distress, depression, anxiety and fear must also be improved. Trials including measures of psychological factors have shown that exercise benefits psychological factors e.g., fear avoidance.[63, 64]

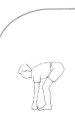

Reducing pain for people with persistent LBP	
12. Strengthening exercises are more effective than no active intervention in improving psychological status agree mid disagree 60% 24% 16%	**For** We need to enforce the message to remain active and emphasise that people's backs are strong structures that are not easily damaged. Extrapolating from sports science there ought to be a good feeling for people focusing on strengthening exercises If mobilising exercises can ↓ pain and ↑ function why would anybody think that they do not also ↑ psychological status more effectively than no active intervention. Physiotherapists tend to target ↓ pain and ↑ function but pain related distress, depression, anxiety and fear must also be improved. Trials including measures of psychological factors [64] [63] have shown that exercise benefits psychological factors e.g., fear avoidance. **Against / mid** Trials of exercise programmes demonstrating psychological benefit have typically been aerobic / circuit type group exercise. Is it really possible to generalise from these that a subgroup of exercises such as strengthening exercises will produce similar effects?
13. Unsupervised walking is more effective than no active intervention in improving psychological status agree mid disagree 84% 12% 4%	No discussion, consensus reached in the first round questionnaire
14. Organised aerobic exercises are more effective than no active intervention in improving psychological status agree mid disagree 96% 4% 0%	No discussion, consensus reached in the first round questionnaire
15. Generalised exercises are more effective than no active intervention in improving psychological status agree mid disagree 88% 12% 0%	No discussion, consensus reached in the first round questionnaire
16. Core stability exercises are more effective than no active intervention in improving psychological status agree mid disagree 32% 52% 16%	**For** Skilled practitioners are required and the emphasis needs to be on teaching the control and enabling ↑ function **Against / mid** Experience suggests that psychological status ↑ more with generalised mobilising and strengthening exercises and advice to continue exercising. Focusing on core stability exercises may be detrimental if not integrated with functional activities People may become fearful of undertaking normal activities especially bending and lifting without setting their abdominals first If the focus is purely to 'activate' the stability muscles, then it could be detrimental. Fear avoidance can be ↑ where people believe their spine is unstable.

Reducing pain for people with persistent LBP	
17. Hydrotherapy exercises are more effective than no active intervention in improving psychological status agree mid disagree 60% 36% 4%	**For** The experience of BackCare self-help groups is that people enjoy their sessions which are social as well as therapeutic with much laughter. People can move in the warm water in a way that is impossible on dry land and this increases confidence and well being Enjoyment increases confidence, mood and compliance. A workplace questionnaire of 110 people with persistent LBP found 82% reported ↑ well being after a course of hydrotherapy **Against / mid** The problem with hydrotherapy is maintaining the exercise longer-term but this can be addressed by people with persistent LBP participating in land based programmes in parallel with their hydrotherapy
18. McKenzie exercises are more effective than no active intervention in improving psychological status agree mid disagree 52% 24% 24%	**For** McKenzie exercises are about empowerment, self-efficacy, confronting pain and ↓ fear avoidance behaviours thus ↑ psychological status is indirectly targeted A trial indicated significant decrease in Beck Depression score where participants were matched in terms of their direction preference and their exercise programme[151] McKenzie exercises must be more effective than 'no active intervention because an active intervention empowers people to take control of their problem etc. **But** It does not have to be McKenzie exercises. A structured programme focussing on ↑ function and ↑ self management is likely to be effective Practitioner expertise and patient choice seems to be a factor **Against / mid** Few good quality studies have measured fear avoidance but there is stronger data on ↓ anxiety and ↓ depression.

Summary of additional email discussion

In parallel with the iCSP discussion some general points were discussed by email. All members of the nominal consensus group were copied into this.

Discussion
I am surprised that most people in the consensus group agree that strengthening exercises, mobilising exercises, and hydrotherapy exercises influence psychological status but they are less inclined to believe that McKenzie exercises and core stability exercises affect psychological status. It seems to me that **it would be extremely likely that these specific and credible forms of exercise would have a positive psychological effect especially when they are taught by specialists and with conviction.**
We have consensus evidence (76%, first round) that unsupervised walking improves function, and consensus evidence (84%, first round) that unsupervised walking improves psychological status. Surely if we can recommend unsupervised walking for both of these outcomes we must be able to recommend credible exercise programmes designed and delivered by specialists?
I feel we should all carefully consider the statements we have been asked to agree or disagree with. They all relate to comparing the intervention with 'no active intervention'. **It is really difficult for me to understand how anyone can disagree with any of the statements.**

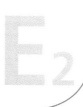

Discussion

Also looking to other guidelines the general advice is movement and activity. Disagreement with the statements seems difficult. Does choice of exercise come down to resources, practitioner speciality and patient choice etc?
Yes. To a large extent it will depend on **resources** and **special interest of the practitioner** more than **patient choice**. I am copying in the European Guidelines[6] recommendations on exercise which summarises my opinion: *We recommend supervised exercise therapy as a first-line treatment in the management of chronic low back pain.* *We advocate the use of exercise programmes that do not require expensive training machines. The use of a cognitive-behavioural approach, in which graded exercises are performed, using exercise quotas, appears to be advisable. Group exercise constitutes an attractive option for treating large numbers of patients at low cost. We do not give recommendations on the specific type of exercise to be undertaken (strengthening/muscle conditioning, aerobic, McKenzie, flexion exercises, etc.). The latter may be best determined by the exercise-preferences of both the patient and therapist.[6]*
I also find it very difficult to disagree with any of the consensus questions i.e., comparing an activity with no active intervention. **I strongly agree that it is better for a person with persistent LBP to be active than non-active.** I think that **the particular type of exercise that is right for any individual depends on their presentation.** If they are stiff then they need mobilising exercises. If they have muscle weakness they need strengthening. If there is functional loss they need mobilising, strengthening and functional exercises. If there are psychological barriers (e.g., yellow or blue flags) then these need to be carefully addressed through a CBT (cognitive behavioural therapy) approach or liaison with the workplace. If we answer 'yes' and come to a consensus on all the questions set will the guidelines be of any use in choosing a particular intervention for an individual? We need to consider **grading, patient preference** and a **CBT approach**. We need to stress that physiotherapy intervention must be based on a thorough **physical and functional assessment.** I am not convinced that the exercise preference of the therapist should be a factor.

Discussion

My experience also supports the comments that relate to the European Guidelines above.[6]

Group exercise classes have worked extremely well using low cost equipment. Focus groups of people who have attended classes identified four main themes:
The value of peer support
People continued to exercise following the programme
People's confidence about their condition improved
People were empowered i.e., they needed less medical help at subsequent recurrences.

I agree with:
the statement from the European guidelines
the statement about matching exercises to individual patient assessment
the importance of both therapist and patient preferences.

I agree with the statement from the European guidelines. I also think that **both physiotherapist's and people with persistent LBP's confidence and fears** are a factor.

Following this last comment one of the main purposes of exercise should be to overcome fear of movement or activity where this is a problem.

I'm happy that, assuming a degree of therapist skill is involved, we can answer yes to all questions.

But questions remain:
do all categories of exercise benefit all categories of outcome?
what is the effect of the psychology behind the application?
E.g., there is no evidence that hydrotherapy exercises relieve chronic LBP. I was happy re-visit my initial thoughts and agree that people with LBP experience both improved well being and improved function, I could not agree that hydrotherapy was likely to reduce pain. I answered 'neither agree nor disagree' to a couple of questions.

The results of work place audits that I have carried out support the notion that **therapist skills and ability are reflected in the outcomes achieved.**

If all forms of exercise are beneficial does this matter if a therapist has preferences?

The NHS is committed to improved patient choice and perhaps **many people with persistent LBP feel that they should choose according to their own beliefs.** Taking this into account will make a difference to the wording of our recommendations.

I like the European wording but wonder if this is because I have read the text. Does it look a bit vague to those who haven't read the text?

I would like to state again that I agree with all the statements. It is quite clear to me that exercise and activity, in any form, is better than no activity. This is in every respect (including or perhaps particularly for its effect on well being and psychological status) for people with chronic LBP.

For **unsupervised walking psychosocial factors may adversely affect compliance** with this; **it shouldn't be recommended as a form of treatment.** I nearly always recommend walking but with **advice on pacing** etc.

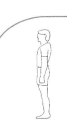

Discussion
I completely agree. In my opinion, **doing something will always be better than doing nothing!** **Also, psychosocial factors are likely to affect compliance with any form of activity, not just unsupervised walking**
I find it very difficult to belief there is disagreement over the usefulness of specific or unstructured regular exercise, rather than doing nothing! It is well known and proven that regular exercise has a positive effect on mild to moderate depression. Multiple international guidelines have repeatedly been unable to endorse many specific treatments but have recommended activity and exercise of a non-specific nature. Specific exercise delivered by a confident and experienced therapist are likely to be more effective.
I agree with those strongly in favour of recommending activity of all types suggested.
I genuinely believe that doing something is preferable to doing nothing at all, both for the treatment effects and the non-specific treatment effects.

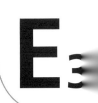

Appendix E3

Exercise for people with persistent low back pain (LBP)

Second round: after iCSP discussion

Please click to mark **one box only** for each question below.
As before, use all your **knowledge** and **experience** (clinical, research, service user) and the **evidence review**.

However, for this round, consider also **how your peers voted in the first round** (the percentage of respondents who marked each box in the first round is indicated below each response box), **how you voted in the first round**, and the **iCSP discussion** for each question.

Statement	Agree	Neither agree nor disagree	Disagree
Reducing pain for people with persistent LBP			
Mobilising exercises are more effective than no active intervention in reducing pain	☐ 60%	☐ 24%	☐ 16%
Unsupervised walking is more effective than no active intervention in reducing pain	☐ 56%	☐ 24%	☐ 20%
Core stability exercises are more effective than no active intervention in reducing pain	☐ 56%	☐ 24%	☐ 20%
Hydrotherapy exercises are more effective than no active intervention in reducing pain	☐ 52%	☐ 32%	☐ 16%
Improving function for people with persistent LBP			
Mobilising exercises are more effective than no active intervention in improving function	☐ 64%	☐ 28%	☐ 8%
Core stability exercises are more effective than no active intervention in improving function	☐ 72%	☐ 16%	☐ 12%
Hydrotherapy exercises are more effective than no active intervention in improving function	☐ 64%	☐ 28%	☐ 8%
McKenzie exercises are more effective than no active intervention in improving function	☐ 60%	☐ 24%	☐ 16%
Improving psychological status for people with persistent LBP			
Mobilising exercises are more effective than no active intervention in improving psychological status	☐ 56%	☐ 32%	☐ 12%
Strengthening exercises are more effective than no active intervention in improving psychological status	☐ 60%	☐ 24%	☐ 16%
Core stability exercises are more effective than no active intervention in improving psychological status	☐ 32%	☐ 52%	☐ 16%
Hydrotherapy exercises are more effective than no active intervention in improving psychological status	☐ 60%	☐ 36%	☐ 4%
McKenzie exercises are more effective than no active intervention in improving psychological status	☐ 52%	☐ 24%	☐ 24%

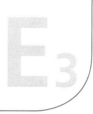

Either email completed form, **by Thursday 19th January 2006**, to Susan Williams at williamss@csp.org.uk or return hard copy to:

Susan Williams, Administrator (R & CE Unit),
The Chartered Society of Physiotherapy,
14 Bedford Row, London, WC1R 4ED.

For your information

We achieved consensus (75% or more agreement) to 5 questions in the first round:

- strengthening exercises improve function
- unsupervised walking improves function
- unsupervised walking improves psychological status
- organised aerobic exercises improve psychological status
- general exercises improve psychological status.

These questions have been removed from this second round questionnaire.

The next stages in developing these guidelines

The guideline development group will make recommendations, for both practice and research, based on the evidence review and the outcome of this consensus exercise.

Thank your help in producing these guidelines!

Note to readers

The question:

Hydrotherapy exercises are more effective than no active intervention in improving function

was included in this questionnaire but there is research evidence for this (section 4.8). The reason is that the research evidence was added to the systematic review **after** this questionnaire was sent out. The research evidence took precedence over the nominal group consensus evidence hence the latter was discarded.

Appendix E4

Summary of consensus results

Statement	% Agree	% Neither agree nor disagree	% Disagree
Reducing pain for people with persistent LBP			
Mobilising exercises are more effective than no active intervention in reducing pain	60	24	16
(second round)	83	9	9
Unsupervised walking is more effective than no active intervention in reducing pain	56	24	20
(second round)	74	17	9
Core stability exercises are more effective than no active intervention in reducing pain	56	24	20
(second round)	74	17	8
Hydrotherapy exercises are more effective than no active intervention in reducing pain	52	32	16
(second round)	83	4	13
Improving function for people with persistent LBP			
Mobilising exercises are more effective than no active intervention in improving function	64	28	8
(second round)	91	4	4
Strengthening exercises are more effective than no active intervention in improving function	80	8	12
Unsupervised walking is more effective than no active intervention in improving function	76	24	0
Core stability exercises are more effective than no active intervention in improving function	72	16	12
(second round)	83	13	4
Hydrotherapy exercises are more effective than no active intervention in improving function	64	28	8
(second round)	87	9	4
McKenzie exercises are more effective than no active intervention in improving function	60	24	16
(second round)	87	13	0
Improving psychological status for people with persistent LBP			
Mobilising exercises are more effective than no active intervention in improving psychological status	56	32	12
(second round)	83	13	4

Statement	% Agree	% Neither agree nor disagree	% Disagree
Strengthening exercises are more effective than no active intervention in improving psychological status	60	24	16
(second round)	87	9	4
Unsupervised walking is more effective than no active intervention in improving psychological status	84	12	4
Organised aerobic exercises are more effective than no active intervention in improving psychological status	96	4	0
Combined exercises are more effective than no active intervention in improving psychological status	88	12	0
Core stability exercises are more effective than no active intervention in improving psychological status	32	52	16
(second round)	61	35	4
Hydrotherapy exercises are more effective than no active intervention in improving psychological status	60	36	4
(second round)	83	9	9
McKenzie exercises are more effective than no active intervention in improving psychological status	52	24	24
(second round)	83	17	0

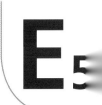

Appendix E5

Summary of the GDG discussion that led to the research recommendations

This gives a flavour of the discussion that began at the GDG meeting of 9th February 2006 and continued by email until publication of these guidelines. All members of the GDG were copied into the email discussion.

Discussion at the GDG meeting of 9th February 2006
Ideas for important research areas that were put forward at this meeting: • Does outcome vary for specific subgroups i.e., those with different expectations or levels of psychological distress? Highlighted as the key research question. • Patient choice • Predicting outcomes • Return to work • Investigation as to whether particular exercises really do what they say the doHow does exercise work? • Evaluation of unsupervised walking programmes • The effect of Psychological status on outcome • Patient Expectations • Which is best, group or individual treatment? It was agreed that this list of research areas would form the basis of the first draft of the research recommendations. The next stage of developing these into the final agreed recommendations would take place by email.
From this list a draft of the research recommendations was made and this was modified by GDG discussion by email between 11th February and the GDG meeting on 21st March 2006 It was recognised that attention to detail was extremely important and there was a great detail of discussion about the precise wording of the recommendations and this cannot be represented here. However a flavour of some of the major points gives an idea about how the final form of the research recommendations was reached.
We need to expand the section on sub-grouping of people with persistent LBP.

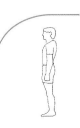

There needs to be more discussion of the methods.

As is the case with most areas of research, you could distinguish two phases in the process of evaluating the effectiveness of an intervention, and each of these phases has slightly different methodology.

The first phase is about developing a new intervention. In this case a small group of subjects is often sufficient and the results are used to improve the intervention. Once the intervention gives promising results, the second phase starts. In this phase it is important to reproduce the results of the first studies in a larger trial, often a multi-centre clinical trial with rigid methodological criteria. Only results of this kind of study can form a solid basis for recommendations for clinical practice. Theoretically these recommendations can also be based on a series of smaller studies, but it has proved challenging to some individual studies due to the variation in interventions, subjects and methodology.

The nature of back pain is not helpful, non-specific low back pain contains a wide range of patients. It is important to realise that back pain is a symptom that has some underlying (in many cases unknown) physiological, anatomical and/or psychological mechanism. It is possible that certain interventions might only benefit a subgroup of patients with back pain, since each intervention interacts with a certain physiological, anatomical and/or psychological system or pathway. One way of exploring this is by studying potential differences in those who responded well to the programme with those who fare less well. Such a comparison should go further than the criteria used to date (e.g., age, gender, duration of complaints, severity of complaints, sick leave). An interesting factor that has been explored in recent years is fear of movement and fear-avoidance behaviour.

At the same time, this huge variation in back pain might explain why many (especially smaller) trials fail to show statistically and clinically significant results. Designing larger, more powerful trials or limiting the variation by trying to apply sub-classification criteria could solve this.

At the teleconference the issue of sub-groups and classification of back pain was flagged as a key issue, thus the key research question is:
> Are there identifiable sub-groups of the back pain population who respond best to specific exercises?

If this is the most important issue then subsidiary research questions relate to exploring the links between assessment, classification, treatment and outcomes; they not necessarily RCTs.

I think one other point needs to come out a bit stronger in our research recommendations and that is:
> It is no use having 'standard physiotherapy' as a treatment arm in any RCT if that intervention is not further specified.

I think it is more a problem in RCTs designed by non-physiotherapists where physiotherapy is a control intervention. Between brackets they then give the various modalities used (e.g., electro-therapy, exercise, manual therapy etc.) but that is all the information that the reader gets. The overall conclusion is then that intervention X is more/less effective than physiotherapy (and that becomes the headline in press releases/newspaper articles etc).

I am not a fan of using 'standard physiotherapy' in RCTs, but I can see the benefit of this in some cases, but more description should always be given.

I still do not think the research recommendations make clear the importance of identifying sub-groups and testing out interventions on these subgroups, which I think most seem to think is an important research direction. For instance:

- reliability studies are needed to identify reproducible methods of assessment / classification
- cohort studies are needed to identify useful sub-groups that have prognostic validity
- sub-group trials need to be conducted that seek to identify the most effective intervention.

There are further questions I think should be included:

- Are specific exercises more effective than non-specific exercises?
- Do you have to treat psychological problems directly to affect them?

Discussion at the GDG meeting of 21st March 2006

At this meeting the GDG were generally happy with the research recommendations and just two changes were made as follows:

- Unsupervised walking became unsupervised exercise (walking, cycling, swimming) in order to stress the value of a wider range of exercises
- A question about the safety of exercise was not felt to be a priority and was omitted from the final version
- Other minor changes were made to the wording of some recommendations.

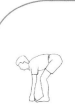

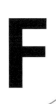

Appendix F

Glossary and abbreviations

Term	Meaning
Black flags	The actual barriers preventing a person from returning to work, these are called the organisational obstacles to recovery.
Blue flags	A person's perception of the barriers preventing them from returning to work.
Cauda equina syndrome	Injury to the spinal roots emerging from the lower end of the spinal cord below the level of the second lumbar vertebrae causing a range of symptoms including impaired bowel and bladder control, sexual dysfunction, weakness in the legs, pain.
Chartered Society of Physiotherapy (CSP)	The professional body for physiotherapists in the UK.
Chronic low back pain	Persistent symptoms lasting more than six weeks
Cochrane Collaboration	An international non-profit and independent organisation producing and disseminating systematic reviews of healthcare interventions. The Cochrane Database of Systematic Reviews and other useful databases are published on The Cochrane Library.
Cognitive intervention	A talking (hands off) therapy conducted by a trained therapist that identifies and modifies negative patterns of thinking, changes emotional responses and behaviour.
Consensus	General agreement.
Controlled trial	A prospective, experimental study that compares a group of people that are given a therapy of interest with at least one other control group, who are usually given standard therapy, a placebo/sham therapy or no treatment.
Control group	The study participants that have not received the experimental intervention. Coping strategies A person's style, or strategy for coping with situations that involve psychological stress or threat.
Cost-effective	Extent to which funds spent to improve health and well-being reduce overall cost of care. Continuing professional development (CPD) The systematic maintenance, improvement and broadening of knowledge and skills and the development of personal qualities necessary for the execution of professional duties throughout the practitioner's working life.
CT (Computed Tomography) scan	A special radiographic technique that uses a computer to assimilate multiple X-ray images into a 2 dimensional cross-sectional image.
Discitis	Inflammation of an intervertebral disk or disk space which may lead to disk erosion.
Disseminate	Disperse or spread knowledge.

Effect size	A way of quantifying the difference between an intervention group and a control group. Generally the larger the effect size the greater the effect of an intervention. Various formulae are used e.g., $$\frac{\text{mean of the intervention group} - \text{mean of the control group}}{\text{standard deviation}}$$
Electrotherapy	The use of electricity to treat disease.
Epidemiology	The study of the prevalence and spread of disease in a community.
Evidence tables	A table demonstrating details of research findings.
Fear avoidance	Avoidance of activity resulting from a person's belief that the experience of pain will lead to further damage and/ or (re)injury.
Guideline development group (GDG)	Team of clinical experts, research methodologists, patient representatives and administrators who worked together to produce these guidelines.
Hydrotherapy	Physiotherapy treatment immersed in a pool incorporating the physical principles of water.
iCSP (interactive CSP)	A web-site that enables members of the CSP to keep up to date with professional interests, to interact with peers and to access a large database of practical knowledge and resources.
Implement	A deliberate action performed to achieve a goal, such as a plan to facilitate the use of these guidelines in clinical practice.
Manipulative Therapy / manual therapy	The passive, sometimes forceful movement of bones, joints and soft tissues carried out by trained therapists, usually to relieve pain, reduce joint stiffness or correct deformity. Manipulation and manual mobilisation are forms of manipulative or manual therapy.
Manipulation	A high velocity, small amplitude thrust performed by the therapist at the end of the available range of movement that is not under the control of the patient.
Manual mobilisation	Small rhythmical oscillations, or sustained pressure, by the therapist within the range of movement that can be resisted by the patient if the procedure becomes too painful.
Massage	Systematic rubbing of the skin and deeper tissues. Massage helps to improve circulation, prevent scarring in injured tissues, relax muscle spasms, improve muscle tone and reduce swelling.
McKenzie method	A concept of assessment and treatment of the spine. A musculoskeletal approach to management.
Median	The middle value in a series of numbers, a statistical term.
Motor control	The ability of the central nervous system to direct and control movement
MRI (Magnetic Resonance Imaging)	Magnetic fields and radio frequencies are used to produce clear images of body tissue.
National Health Service (NHS)	The government led health system in the UK.

National Institute of Clinical Excellence	An independent organisation funded by the NHS responsible for providing national guidance on the use of treatments and the provision of care in the UK.
Neurological	Relating to the nervous system
Non specific low back pain	Low back pain not attributed to recognisable, known specific pathology (e.g., infection, tumour, osteoporosis, ankylosing spondylitis, fracture, inflammatory process, radicular syndrome or cauda equina syndrome).
Osteoarthritis	A degenerative joint disease where the primary problem is change in structure of cartilage and bone, rather than an inflammatory synovitis.
Osteoporosis	A metabolic bone disease resulting from low bone mass (osteopenia) due to excessive bone resorption. Sufferers are prone to bone fractures from relatively minor trauma.
Outcome	The result of treatment on the patient or client
Outcome measure	A validated test or scale for measuring a particular outcome of interest in order to assess the effectiveness of a therapy or service.
Palpate	Examine medically by touch.
PEDro (Physiotherapy Evidence Database)	Database of controlled clinical trials and systematic reviews on the effectiveness of physiotherapy interventions.
Physical mixed methods	A physiotherapy modality that is not manual e.g., electrotherapy and ice.
Physical therapy	This term is used broadly to include non-medical 'hands on' treatment and includes physiotherapy in addition to osteopathy etc.
Physiotherapy interventions	Specific treatments used by chartered physiotherapists, in partnership with patients, to work towards an agreed goal e.g., an exercise programme designed to reduce pain.
Placebo	An inactive treatment made to look and feel the same as an active treatment. It is used for a control group in a RCT so that it is possible to measure the outcome of the intervention being investigated.
Power (of an RCT)	Where the power is high there is a high chance of a statistically significant result (where this would be a true result). e.g., 80% power means an 80% chance of ending up with a statistically significant result (specifically, a p value of less than 5%). By convention 80% is an acceptable level of power.
PRODIGY guidance	Source of clinical knowledge based on the best available evidence about common conditions and symptoms managed in primary care. Produced by the Sowerby Centre for Health Informatics at Newcastle.
Prognosis	Prediction of the patient's outcome or the course their recovery will take. Prospective study A trial in which patients are recruited according to the criteria laid down in the protocol. Patients may be treated with a new intervention and followed up afterwards to assess the effect of treatment. Clinical trials are prospective studies.
Psychosocial factors	Combination of psychological and social factors.
Quality of life	Self report defining the quality of a person's life usually related to physical, mental, social, and role functioning in addition to perception of well-being.
Quasi-	Almost, seemingly.

Quasi-experimental	Quasi-experimental research is characterised by less control than true experimental research, and this lesser degree of control of the experimental situation is achieved either with a single subject group, whereby subjects act as their own controls, or by using multiple groups to which subjects are not randomly assigned.
Radicular pain	Pain experienced in a particular dermatome (an area of skin supplied by sensory nerve fibres of a single nerve root) due to pressure on the nerve root.
Randomised controlled trial (RCT)	A clinical trial comparing two or more groups of people, from a given population, who are given different interventions. They are allocated to groups at random (see randomisation).
Randomised	Assigning participants in a randomised controlled trial to treatment groups on a random basis in an attempt to ensure the groups are balanced.
Red flags	Factors that may indicate serious pathology.
Reflective practice	Self-awareness and critical analysis of an experience in order to learn from it and improve clinical practice.
Reliability	The extent to which the results of a study can be reproduced if the study is carried out again exactly as reported.
Self-efficacy	A person's belief in their ability to achieve a specific goal e.g., returning to normal function regardless of persistent LBP.
Sham group	A group receiving a dummy procedure made to look and feel like an active therapy. See placebo.
Short-wave diathermy	High frequency, short-wave electrical currents with wavelengths of 3 to 30 metres, used to provide heat deep into the body.
Somatic	The body, as distinguished from the mind or psyche.
Spondylitis	Inflammation of the vertebrae.
Spondylolysthesis	Forward displacement of one vertebra on the bone below it. Most commonly seen at L5/S1 level. The degree of spondylolisthesis is determined by the distance the slipped vertebra travels on its lower counterpart.
Standard deviation	A measure of the spread of data i.e., how much the values vary from each other or the spread of data around the mean.
Statistically significant	The results of a study have probably not occurred by chance and a true difference has been observed.
Systematic review	A scientific method for collecting, appraising, synthesising and communicating all the available research on a particular topic.
Thoracic	Pertaining to the chest.
Thoracic spine	Comprises of 12 vertebrae between the cervical and lumbar spines and providing attachment for the ribs.
Traction	A manual or motorised electrical modality to distract joint surfaces. It can either be intermittent or a sustained force.
Ultrasound	The diagnostic or therapeutic use of high-frequency sound waves to produce heat.
Validity	The extent to which a research finding is accurate and measures what it purports to measure.

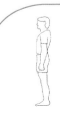

Visual analogue scale (VAS)	A scale used to provide a quantitative measure of a subjective outcome, such as pain. The scale is usually a 10cm line with definitions at either end, e.g., "no pain" at 0cm and "worse pain ever felt" at the 10cm end. The distance from 0cm to the mark on the line indicated by the patient is his or her pain score.
Yellow flags	Psychological and sociological factors that increase the risk of developing or perpetuating long-term disability and work loss associated with low back pain.

Bibliography

The following resources were used in compiling this glossary:

American Medical Massage Association (AMMA). 2006. Available from: http://www.americanmedicalmassage.com/ (accessed 4th April 2006)

Bottomley JM, editor (2002) **Quick reference dictionary for physical therapy (2nd ed.)** New Jersey: Slack Incorporated.

British School of Osteopathy. What is Osteopathy? Available from: http://bso.ac.uk/mm1aost.htm (accessed 29th November 2006).

Churchill's illustrated medical dictionary (1989) New York: Churchill Livingstone.

Domholdt, E (1993) **Physical therapy research: principles and applications**, London: Harcourt Brace.

Hutchinson DR. Dictionary of clinical research (2002) (3rd ed.) Richmond: Brookwood Medical Publications Ltd.

Hyperdictionary. Available from: http://www.hyperdictionary.com/ (Accessed 11 May 2004)

Khan KS, ter Riet G, Glanville J, Sowden A, Kleijnen J, editors. **Undertaking systematic reviews of research on effectiveness. CRD Report 4. 2nd ed**. York: NHS Centre for Reviews and Dissemination; 2001.

Mosby's medical, nursing, & allied health dictionary. 6th ed. St. Louis, Missouri: Mosby; 2002.

National Electronic Library for Health. Dictionaries and Internet searching. Available from: http://www.nelh.nhs.uk/directories.asp (Accessed 11 May 2004).

Pearsall, J editor (2002) **Concise Oxford English Dictionary** (10th ed) Oxford: Oxford University Press.

Porter S (2005) **Dictionary of Physiotherapy.** Elsevier: London.

University of Newcastle upon Tyne. On-line medical dictionary. Available from: http://cancerweb.ncl.ac.uk/cgi-bin/omd?action=Home&query= (Accessed 11 May 2004).

van Tulder, M et al (2004) **European Guidelines for the Management of Acute Nonspecific Low Back Pain in Primary Care**, COST B13 Working Group on Guidelines for the Management of Acute Low Back Pain in Primary Care.

G

Appendix G

Links to other guidelines

Readers may find the following links to other guidelines for back pain useful.

Airaksinen O, Bronx JI, Cedraschi C, Hildebrandt J, Klaber Moffett J, Kovacs F, et al. European guidelines for the management of chronic non-specific low back pain. European commission, research directorate general 2004. Available from: www.backpaineurope.org/web/html/wg2_results.html (accessed 27th November 2006)[6]

PRODIGY. PRODIGY guidance - back pain - lower. Department of Health 2005. Available from: www.prodigy.nhs.uk/back_pain_lower (accessed 27th November 2006)[20]

Arthritis and musculoskeletal alliance. Standards of care for people with back pain. Arthritis and musculoskeletal alliance 2004. Available from: http://www.arma.uk.net/care.html (accessed 27th November 2006)[21]

Clinical Standards Advisory Group (CSAG). Back pain. London: HMSO; 1994. Danish Institute for Health Technology Assessment. Frequency, Management and Prevention from an HTA perspective[22]

Danish Institute for Health Technology Assessment 1999. Available from: www.sst.dk/Applikationer/ cemtv/publikationer/docs/Low-back%20pain/default.html (accessed 27th November 2006)[169]

The European Agency for Safety and Health at Work (there are a number of useful documents here). http://uk.osha.eu.int/good_practice/msd.stm

Bekkering GE, Hendriks HJM, Koes BW, Oostendorp RAB, Ostelo RWJG, Thomassen JMC, et al. Dutch physiotherapy guidelines for low back pain. Physiotherapy 2003;89[2]:82-96[170]

Institute for Clinical Systems Improvement. Health Care Guideline: Adult Low Back Pain. Institute for Clinical Systems Improvement 2006. Available from: http://www.icsi.org/knowledge/detail. asp?catID=29&itemID=149 (accessed 30th November 2006)[171]

Philadelphia Panel. Philadelphia panel evidence-based clinical practice guidelines on selected rehabilitation interventions for neck pain. Phys Ther 2001;81[10]:1701-17[172]

Waddell G, Burton K. Occupational health guidelines for the management of low back pain at work - evidence review. Faculty of Occupational Medicine. 2000. Available from: www.facoccmed.ac.uk/library/ index.jsp?ref=383 (accessed 27th November 2006)[173]

New Zealand Guidelines Group. New Zealand acute low back pain guide. New Zealand Guidelines Group 2004. Available from: www.nzgg.org.nz/index.cfm?fuseaction=fuseaction_10&fusesubaction=docs&doc umentID=22 (accessed 27th November 2006)[174]

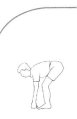

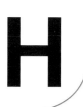

Appendix H

Outcome measures used in the quality RCTs

Analysis of the outcome measures used for pain, function and psychological status was derived (Donchin,[45] Klaber Moffett,[58] Mannion,[56] McIlveen,[72] Petersen,[48] Torstensen,[55] UK BEAM[63, 64]) were larger, higher in methodological quality and included robust statistical analysis.

The analysis here considers the outcome measures used in these trials. The GDG concluded that the measures were generally high in validity and reliability and relevant to the context of these guidelines. Further, many of the measures are those recommended for use by the GDG (section 3.7).

Table 1: measuring pain

Outcome measure Used	Trials used this measure	GDG comment on the validity, reliability and relevance of the measures
The Visual Analogue Scale (VAS) for pain intensity	Mannion[56] Torstensen[55]	A measure with good validity and reliability that is recommended by the GDG for use with people with persistent LBP (section 3.7). For details see: http://www.csp.org.uk/director/effectivepractice/outcomemeasures/database.cfm?item_id=570119BFE46871734E078C4CEB1F66D5
The McGill Pain Questionnaire	McIlveen[72]	A relevant measure with good validity, reliability and relevance. For details see: http://www.csp.org.uk/director/effectivepractice/outcomemeasures/database.cfm?item_id=57011D40E00239D15CF972C25CED9774
Patient reports or patient diaries	Donchin[45] Klaber Moffett[48] Petersen[48]	Patient reports are reliable evidence where the methodology is sound.
Manniche's LBP Rating Scale (MRS)	Petersen[48]	This scale is a multidimensional and specific to back pain that strongly correlates with the Roland-Morris disability questionnaire (RDQ) and this suggests that it is likely to be valid and reliable. To the GDG's knowledge it has not be used in an English language version.
The von Korff Scale	UK BEAM[63, 64]	A relevant measure with sound validity and reliability for pain in people with spinal cord injury (Raichle, 2006 #336).

Table 2: measuring function

The Oswestry Disability Index (ODI)	Donchin[45] McIlveen[72]	A measure with good validity and reliability that is recommended by the GDG for use with people with persistent LBP (section 3.7). For details see: http://www.csp.org.uk/director/effectivepractice/outcomemeasures/database.cfm?item_id=57011DC7E1A1B0DF9335700BCF335C84 or Fairbank 2000[33]
The Roland-Morris Disability Questionnaire (RDQ)	Klaber Moffett[58] Mannion[56] UK BEAM[63, 64]	A measure with good validity and reliability that is recommended by the GDG for use with people with persistent LBP (section 3.7). For details see: http://www.csp.org.uk/director/effectivepractice/outcomemeasures/database.cfm?item_id=57011DCF90E235E91BF2E6F25CAB2E5A or Roland 2000[32]
The Modified von Korff Scale	UK BEAM[63, 64]	A relevant measure with sound validity and reliability.
A measure of 15 activities of daily living	Petersen[48]	The GDG strongly suggest the use of standardised outcome measures. However no Ib evidence was derived from this part of Petersen's study because the evidence in terms of function was inconclusive.

Table 3: measuring psychological status

The Fear Avoidance Beliefs Questionnaire (FABQ)	Klaber Moffett[58] Mannion[56] UK BEAM[63, 64]	A measure with good validity and reliability that is recommended by the GDG for use with people with persistent LBP (section 3.7). For details see: http://www.csp.org.uk/director/effectivepractice/outcomemeasures/database.cfm?item_id=57011CBEA9EF7AA1A8A07D621E3BBEE0 or Waddell 1993[38]
The Back Beliefs Questionnaire	Mannion[56] UK BEAM[63, 64]	A measure with good validity and reliability that is recommended by the GDG for use with people with persistent LBP (section 3.7). For details see: 1995[39]

References

1. Hammond R, Mead J. Identifying national priorities for physical therapy clinical guideline development. In: 14th International WCPT Congress. 7 - 12th June 2003; Barcelona, Spain: The World Conferederation for Physical Therapy; 2003.

2. Croft PR, Macfarlane GJ, Papageorgiou AC, Thomas E, Silman AJ. Outcome of low back pain in general practice: a prospective study. BMJ 1998;316(7141):1356-9.

3. Hestbaek L, Leboeuf-Yde C, Engberg M, Lauritzen T, Bruun NH, Manniche C. The course of low back pain in a general population. Results from a 5-year prospective study. J Manipulative Physiol Ther 2003;26(4):213-9.

4. Hestbaek L, Leboeuf-Yde C, Manniche C. Low back pain: what is the long-term course? A review of studies of general patient populations. Eur Spine J 2003;12(2):149-65.

5. Burton AK, McClune TD, Clarke RD, Main CJ. Long-term follow-up of patients with low back pain attending for manipulative care: outcomes and predictors. Man Ther 2004;9(1):30-5.

6. Airaksinen O, Bronx JI, Cedraschi C, Hildebrandt J, Klaber Moffett J, Kovacs F, et al. European guidelines for the management of chronic non-specific low back pain. European commission, research directorate general 2004. Available from: www.backpaineurope.org/web/html/wg2_results.html (accessed 27th November 2006)

7. Waddell G. The back pain revolution. 2nd ed. London: Churchill Livingstone; 2004.

8. Field MJ, Lohr KNE. Guidelines for clinical practice: from development to use. Washington DC: National Academy Press; 1992.

9. Scottish Intercollegiate Guidelines Network. Sign 50: A guideline developers' handbook. Scottish Intercollegiate Guidelines Network 2001. Available from: http://www.sign.ac.uk/guidelines/fulltext/50/index.html (accessed 29th November 2006)

10. van Tulder MW, Assendelft WJ, Koes BW, Bouter LM. Method guidelines for systematic reviews in the Cochrane Collaboration Back Review Group for Spinal Disorders. Spine 1997;22(20):2323-30.

11. van Tulder M, Furlan A, Bombardier C, Bouter L. Updated method guidelines for systematic reviews in the cochrane collaboration back review group. Spine 2003;28(12):1290-9.

12. Moore RA, Gavaghan D, Tramer MR, Collins SL, McQuay HJ. Size is everything--large amounts of information are needed to overcome random effects in estimating direction and magnitude of treatment effects. Pain 1998;78(3):209-16.

13. Hemmila HM, Keinanen-Kiukaanniemi SM, Levoska S, Puska P. Does folk medicine work? A randomised clinical trial on patients with prolonged back pain. Arch Phys Med Rehabil 1997;78(6):571-7.

14. Hemmila HM, Keinanen-Kiukaanniemi SM, Levoska S, Puska P. Long-term effectiveness of bone-setting, light exercise therapy, and physiotherapy for prolonged back pain: a randomised controlled trial. J Manipulative Physiol Ther 2002;25(2):99-104.

15. Chartered Society of Physiotherapy. Guidance For Developing Clinical Guidelines. London: Chartered Society of Physiotherapy; 2003.

16. National Institute for Clinical Excellence. Information for National Collaborating Centres and Guideline Development Groups. London: National Institute for Clinical Excellence; 2001.

17. Murphy M, Black N, Lamping D, McKee C, Sanderson C, Askham J. Consensus development methods, and their use in clinical guideline development. Health Technology Assessment 1998. Available from: www.hta.nhsweb.nhs.uk/execsumm/summ203.htm (accessed 28th November 2006)

18. Moore A, Jackson A, Jordan J, Hammersley S, Hill J, Mercer C, et al. Clinical guidelines for the physiotherapy management of whiplash associated disorder. London: The Chartered Society of Physiotherapy; 2005.

19. AGREE Collaboration. AGREE Instrument: Appraisal of guidelines for research and evaluation. The AGREE Collaboration 2001. Available from: www.agreecollaboration.org/instrument/ (accessed 27th November 2006)

20. PRODIGY. PRODIGY guidance - back pain - lower. Department of Health 2005. Available from: www.prodigy.nhs.uk/back_pain_lower (accessed 27th November 2006)

21. Arthritis and musculoskeletal alliance. Standards of care for people with back pain. Arthritis and musculoskeletal alliance 2004. Available from: http://www.arma.uk.net/care.html (accessed 27th November 2006)

22. Clincal Standards Advisory Group (CSAG). Back pain. London: HMSO; 1994.

23. Aina A, May S, Clare H. The centralization phenomenon of spinal symptoms – a systematic review. Man Ther 2004;9(3):134-43.

24. Roberts L, Fraser S, Murphy E. Red flags or red herrings? In: The Society for Back Pain Research. 10th-11th November 2005; University of Warwick; 2005.

25. Harding IJ, Davies E, Buchanan E, Fairbank JT. The symptom of night pain in a back pain triage clinic. Spine 2005;30(17):1985-8.

26. Bartys S, Burton K, Wright I, Mackay C, Watson P, Main C. Organisational obstacles to recovery (black flags) from musculoskeletal disorders. Contemp Ergon 2002:203-210.

27. Coulter A, Ellis J. The quality enhancing interventions project: patient-focused interventions. London: The Health Foundation; 2006.

28. Chartered Society of Physiotherapy. Core Standards of Physiotherapy Practice. London: The Chartered Society of Physiotherapy; 2005.

29. Dworkin RH, Turk DC, Farrar JT, Haythornthwaite JA, Jensen MP, Katz NP, et al. Core outcome measures for chronic pain clinical trials: IMMPACT recommendations. Pain 2005;113(1-2):9-19.

30. Kopec JA, Esdaile JM, Abrahamowicz M, Abenhaim L, Wood-Dauphinee S, Lamping DL, et al. The Quebec Back Pain Disability Scale: conceptualising and development. J Clin Epidemiol 1996;49(2):151-61.

31. Ruta DA, Garratt AM, Wardlaw D, Russell IT. Developing a valid and reliable measure of health outcome for patients with low back pain. Spine 1994;19(17):1887-96.

32. Roland M, Fairbank J. The Roland-Morris Disability Questionnaire and the Oswestry Disability Questionnaire. Spine 2000;25(24):3115-24.

33. Fairbank JC, Pynsent PB. The Oswestry Disability Index. Spine 2000;25(22):2940-52; discussion 2952.

34. Ware JE, Jr., Sherbourne CD. The MOS 36-item short-form health survey (SF-36). I. Conceptual framework and item selection. Med Care 1992;30(6):473-83.

35. Chwastiak LA, Von Korff M. Disability in depression and back pain: evaluation of the World Health Organization Disability Assessment Schedule (WHO DAS II) in a primary care setting. J Clin Epidemiol 2003;56(6):507-14.

36. Anderson KO, Dowds BN, Pelletz RE, Edwards WT, Peeters-Asdourian C. Development and initial validation of a scale to measure self-efficacy beliefs in patients with chronic pain. Pain 1995;63(1):77-84.

37. Main CJ, Wood PL, Hollis S, Spanswick CC, Waddell G. The Distress and Risk Assessment Method. A simple patient classification to identify distress and evaluate the risk of poor outcome. Spine 1992;17(1):42-52.

38. Waddell G, Newton M, Henderson I, Somerville D, Main CJ. A Fear-Avoidance Beliefs Questionnaire (FABQ) and the role of fear-avoidance beliefs in chronic low back pain and disability. Pain 1993;52(2):157-68.

39. Symonds TL, Burton AK, Tillotson KM, Main CJ. Absence resulting from low back trouble can be reduced by psychosocial intervention at the work place. Spine 1995;20(24):2738-45.

40. Woby SR, Roach NK, Urmston M, Watson PJ. Psychometric properties of the TSK-11: a shortened version of the Tampa Scale for Kinesiophobia. Pain 2005;117(1-2):137-44.

41. Pincus T, Williams AC, Vogel S, Field A. The development and testing of the depression, anxiety, and positive outlook scale (DAPOS). Pain 2004;109(1-2):181-8.

42. Deyo RA, Battie M, Beurskens AJ, Bombardier C, Croft P, Koes B, et al. Outcome measures for low back pain research. A proposal for standardized use. Spine 1998;23(18):2003-13.

43. Tritilanunt T, Wajanavisit W. The efficacy of an aerobic exercise and health education programme for treatment of chronic low back pain. J Med Assoc Thai 2001;84 Suppl 2:S528-33.

44. Elnaggar IM, Nordin M, Sheikhzadeh A, Parnianpour M, Kahanovitz N. Effects of spinal flexion and extension exercises on low-back pain and spinal mobility in chronic mechanical low-back pain patients. Spine 1991;16(8):967-72.

45. Donchin M, Woolf O, Kaplan L, Floman Y. Secondary prevention of low-back pain. A clinical trial. Spine 1990;15(12):1317-20.

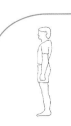

References

46. Martin PR, Rose MJ, Nichols PJ, Russell PL, Hughes IG. Physiotherapy exercises for low back pain: process and clinical outcome. Int Rehabil Med 1986;8(1):34-8.

47. Manniche C, Lundberg E, Christensen I, Bentzen L, Hesselsoe G. Intensive dynamic back exercises for chronic low back pain: a clinical trial. Pain 1991;47(1):53-63.

48. Petersen T, Kryger P, Ekdahl C, Olsen S, Jacobsen S. The effect of McKenzie therapy as compared with that of intensive strengthening training for the treatment of patients with subacute or chronic low back pain: A randomised controlled trial. Spine 2002;27(16):1702-9.

49. Koumantakis GA, Watson PJ, Oldham JA. Trunk muscle stabilisation training plus general exercise versus general exercise only: randomised controlled trial of patients with recurrent low back pain. Phys Ther 2005;85(3):209-25.

50. Rittweger J, Just K, Kautzsch K, Reeg P, Felsenberg D. Treatment of chronic lower back pain with lumbar extension and whole-body vibration exercise: a randomised controlled trial. Spine 2002;27(17):1829-34.

51. Helmhout PH, Harts CC, Staal JB, Candel MJ, de Bie RA. Comparison of a high-intensity and a low-intensity lumbar extensor training programme as minimal intervention treatment in low back pain: a randomised trial. Eur Spine J 2004;13(6):537-47.

52. Roland M, Waddell G, Klaber Moffett J, Burton K, Main C. The Back Book. 2nd ed. Norwich: Stationery Office; 1999.

53. Turner JA, Clancy S, McQuade KJ, Cardenas DD. Effectiveness of behavioral therapy for chronic low back pain: a component analysis. J Consult Clin Psychol 1990;58(5):573-9.

54. Storheim K, Brox JI, Holm I, Koller AK, Bo K. Intensive group training versus cognitive intervention in sub-acute low back pain: short-term results of a single-blind randomised controlled trial. J Rehabil Med 2003;35(3):132-40.

55. Torstensen TA, Ljunggren AE, Meen HD, Odland E, Mowinckel P, Geijerstam S. Efficiency and costs of medical exercise therapy, conventional physiotherapy, and self-exercise in patients with chronic low back pain. A pragmatic, randomised, single-blinded, controlled trial with 1-year follow-up. Spine 1998;23(23):2616-24.

56. Mannion AF, Muntener M, Taimela S, Dvorak J. A randomised clinical trial of three active therapies for chronic low back pain. Spine 1999;24(23):2435-48.

57. Johannsen F, Remvig L, Kryger P, Beck P, Warming S, Lybeck K, et al. Exercises for chronic low back pain: a clinical trial. J Orthop Sports Phys Ther 1995;22(2):52-9.

58. Klaber Moffett J, Torgerson D, Bell Syer S, Jackson D, Llewelyn Phillips H, Farrin A, et al. Randomised controlled trial of exercise for low back pain: clinical outcomes, costs, and preferences. BMJ 1999;319(7205):279-83.

59. Callaghan MJ. Evaluation of a back rehabilitation group for chronic low back pain in an out-patient setting. Physiotherapy 1994;80(10):677-81.

60. Kuukkanen TM, Malkia EA. An experimental controlled study on postural sway and therapeutic exercise in subjects with low back pain. Clin Rehabil 2000;14(2):192-202.

61. Snook SH, Webster BS, McGorry RW, Fogleman MT, McCann KB. The reduction of chronic nonspecific low back pain through the control of early morning lumbar flexion. A randomised controlled trial. Spine 1998;23(23):2601-7.

62. Risch SV, Norvell NK, Pollock ML, Risch ED, Langer H, Fulton M, et al. Lumbar strengthening in chronic low back pain patients. Physiologic and psychological benefits. Spine 1993;18(2):232-8.

63. UK BEAM trial team. United Kingdom back pain exercise and manipulation (UK BEAM) randomised trial: cost effectiveness of physical treatments for back pain in primary care. BMJ 2004;329(7479):1381.

64. UK BEAM trial team. United Kingdom back pain exercise and manipulation (UK BEAM) randomised trial: effectiveness of physical treatments for back pain in primary care. BMJ 2004;329(7479):1377.

65. Gur A, Karakoc M, Cevik R, Nas K, Sarac AJ. Efficacy of low power laser therapy and exercise on pain and functions in chronic low back pain. Lasers Surg Med 2003;32(3):233-8.

66. Jousset N, Fanello S, Bontoux L, Dubus V, Billabert C, Vielle B, et al. Effects of functional restoration versus 3 hours per week physical therapy: a randomised controlled study. Spine 2004;29(5):487-93; discussion 494.

67. Kankaanpaa M, Taimela S, Airaksinen O, Hanninen O. The efficacy of active rehabilitation in chronic low back pain. Effect on pain intensity, self-experienced disability, and lumbar fatigability. Spine 1999;24(10):1034-42.

68. Yozbatiran N, Yildirim Y, Parlak B. Effects of fitness and aquafitness exercises on physical fitness in patients with chronic low back pain. Pain Clin 2004;16(1):35-42.

69. Reilly K, Lovejoy B, Williams R, Roth H. Differences between a supervised and independent strength and conditioning programme with chronic low back syndromes. J Occup Med 1989;31(6):547-50.

70. Shaughnessy M, Caulfield B. A pilot study to investigate the effect of lumbar stabilisation exercise training on functional ability and quality of life in patients with chronic low back pain. Int J Rehabil Res 2004;27(4):297-301.

71. Rasmussen-Barr E, Nilsson-Wikmar L, Arvidsson I. Stabilising training compared with manual treatment in sub-acute and chronic low-back pain. Man Ther 2003;8(4):233-41.

72. McIlveen B, Robertson VJ. A randomised controlled study of the outcome of hydrotherapy for subjects with low back or back and leg pain. Physiotherapy 1998;84(1):17-26.

73. Lindstrom I. A successful intervention programme for patients with subacute low back pain: a randomised study using operant conditioning behavioural approach with special reference to pain, pain behaviour, subjective disability, physical performance, physical work demand. Goteborg: Goteborg University; 1994.

74. Lindstrom I, Ohlund C, Eek C, Wallin L, Peterson LE, Fordyce WE, et al. The effect of graded activity on patients with subacute low back pain: a randomised prospective clinical study with an operant-conditioning behavioural approach. Phys Ther 1992;72(4):279-90; discussion 291-3.

75. Lindstrom I, Ohlund C, Eek C, Wallin L, Peterson LE, Nachemson A. Mobility, strength, and fitness after a graded activity programme for patients with subacute low back pain. A randomised prospective clinical study with a behavioural therapy approach. Spine 1992;17(6):641-52.

76. White AW. Low back pain in men receiving workmen's compensation: a follow-up study. Can Med Assoc J 1969;101(2):61-7.

77. Deyo RA, Walsh NE, Martin DC, Schoenfeld LS, Ramamurthy S. A controlled trial of transcutaneous electrical nerve stimulation (TENS) and exercise for chronic low back pain. N Engl J Med 1990;322(23):1627-34.

78. Frost H, Lamb SE, Klaber Moffett JA, Fairbank JC, Moser JS. A fitness programme for patients with chronic low back pain: 2-year follow-up of a randomised controlled trial. Pain 1998;75(2-3):273-9.

79. Klein RG, Eek BC. Low-energy laser treatment and exercise for chronic low back pain: double-blind controlled trial. Arch Phys Med Rehabil 1990;71(1):34-7.

80. Lidstrom A, Zachrisson M. Physical therapy on low back pain and sciatica. An attempt at evaluation. Scand J Rehabil Med 1970;2(1):37-42.

81. Houben RM, Vlaeyen JW, Peters M, Ostelo RW, Wolters PM, Stomp-van den Berg SG. Health care providers' attitudes and beliefs towards common low back pain: factor structure and psychometric properties of the HC-PAIRS. Clin J Pain 2004;20(1):37-44.

82. Houben RM, Gijsen A, Peterson J, de Jong PJ, Vlaeyen JW. Do health care providers' attitudes towards back pain predict their treatment recommendations? Differential predictive validity of implicit and explicit attitude measures. Pain 2005;114(3):491-8.

83. Daykin AR, Richardson B. Physiotherapists' pain beliefs and their influence on the management of patients with chronic low back pain. Spine 2004;29(7):783-95.

84. Linton SJ, Vlaeyen J, Ostelo R. The back pain beliefs of health care providers: are we fear-avoidant? J Occup Rehabil 2002;12(4):223-32.

85. Rainville J, Carlson N, Polatin P, Gatchel RJ, Indahl A. Exploration of physicians' recommendations for activities in chronic low back pain. Spine 2000;25(17):2210-20.

86. BackCare. A People's Guide to Active Backcare. Teddington: BackCare; 2006.

87. Bekkering GE. Physiotherapy guidelines for low back pain: development, implementation and evaluation. PhD Thesis, Dutch Institute of Allied Health Care and the Institute for Research in Extramural Medicine (EMGO Institute) of the VU University Medical Centre; 2004.

88. Foster NE, Doughty GM. Dissemination and implementation of back pain guidelines: perspectives of

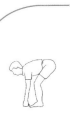

References

musculoskeletal physiotherapists and managers. In: 6th International forum for low back pain research in primary care. May 2003 2003; Linkping, Sweden; 2003.

89. Stevenson K, Lewis M, Hay E. Does physiotherapy management of low back pain change as a result of an evidence-based educational programme? J Eval Clin Pract 2006;12(3):365-75.

90. Mondloch MV, Cole DC, Frank JW. Does how you do depend on how you think you'll do? A systematic review of the evidence for a relation between patients' recovery expectations and health outcomes. CMAJ 2001;165(2):174-9.

91. Thomas E, Croft PR, Paterson SM, Dziedzic K, Hay EM. What influences participants' treatment preference and can it influence outcome? Results from a primary care-based randomised trial for shoulder pain. Br J Gen Pract 2004;54(499):93-6.

92. King M, Nazareth I, Lampe F, Bower P, Chandler M, Morou M, et al. Impact of participant and physician intervention preferences on randomised trials: a systematic review. JAMA 2005;293(9):1089-99.

93. Verbeek J, Sengers MJ, Riemens L, Haafkens J. Patient expectations of treatment for back pain: a systematic review of qualitative and quantitative studies. Spine 2004;29(20):2309-18.

94. Evans DW, Foster NE, Underwood M, Vogel S, Breen AC, Pincus T. Testing the effectiveness of an innovative information package on practitioner reported behaviour and beliefs: the UK Chiropractors, Osteopaths and Musculoskeletal Physiotherapists Low back pain ManagemENT (COMPLeMENT) trial [ISRCTN77245761]. BMC Musculoskelet Disord 2005;6:41.

95. Feuerstein M, Hartzell M, Rogers HL, Marcus SC. Evidence-based practice for acute low back pain in primary care: Patient outcomes and cost of care. Pain 2006;124(1-2):140-49; comment 7-8.

96. Chartered Society of Physiotherapy. Physiotherapy guidelines for the management of osteoporosis – audit pack. London: Chartered Society of Physiotherapy; 2002.

97. National Institute for Clinical Excellence. Princples of Best Practice in Clinical Audit. Oxford: Radclife Medical Press; 2002.

98. Bronfort G, Goldsmith CH, Nelson CF, Boline PD, Anderson AV. Trunk exercise combined with spinal manipulative or NSAID therapy for chronic low back pain: a randomised, observer-blinded clinical trial. J Manipulative Physiol Ther 1996;19(9):570-82.

99. Indahl A, Velund L, Reikeraas O. Good prognosis for low back pain when left untampered: a randomised clinical trial. Spine 1995;20(4):473-7.

100. Jackson DA. How is low back pain managed? Retrospective study of the first 200 patients with low back pain referred to a newly established community-based physiotherapy department. Physiotherapy 2001;87(11):573-81.

101. Lahad A, Malter AD, Berg AO, Deyo RA. The effectiveness of four interventions for the prevention of low back pain. JAMA 1994;272(16):1286-91.

102. van Tulder MW, Koes BW, Bouter LM. Conservative treatment of acute and chronic nonspecific low back pain. A systematic review of randomised controlled trials of the most common interventions. Spine 1997;22(18):2128-56.

103. Klaber Moffett JA, Chase SM, Portek I, Ennis JR. A controlled, prospective study to evaluate the effectiveness of a back school in the relief of chronic low back pain. Spine 1986;11(2):120-2.

104. Airaksinen O, Brox JI, Cedraschi C, Hildebrandt J, Klaber Moffett J, Kovacs F, et al. Chapter 4. European guidelines for the management of chronic nonspecific low back pain. Eur Spine J 2006;15 Suppl 2:S192-300.

105. Hayden JA, van Tulder MW, Malmivaara A, Koes BW. Exercise therapy for treatment of non-specific low back pain. The Cochrane Library 2006;1.

106. Hayden JA, van Tulder MW, Tomlinson G. Systematic review: strategies for using exercise therapy to improve outcomes in chronic low back pain. Ann Intern Med 2005;142(9):776-85.

107. American College of Sports Medicine, Guidelines for exercise testing and prescription. 7th ed: American College of Sports Medicine; 2005.

108. Educational Opportunities Inc. Back Care Programme. Bloomington MN: Educational Opportunities Inc.

109. David Back Clinic. David Back Clinic Treatment Guide. Vantaa: David Back Clinic International; 1994.

110. Kendall PH, Jenkins JM. Exercises for backache: a double-blind controlled trial. Physiotherapy 1968(54):154-157.

111. Manniche C, Hesselsoe G, Bentzen L, Christensen I, Lundberg E. Clinical trial of intensive muscle training for chronic low back pain. Lancet 1988;2(8626-8627):1473-6.

112. Mannion AF, Junge A, Taimela S, Muntener M, Lorenzo K, Dvorak J. Active therapy for chronic low back pain: part 3. Factors influencing self-rated disability and its change following therapy. Spine 2001;26(8):920-9.

113. Taimela S, Harkapaa K. Strength, mobility, their changes, and pain reduction in active functional restoration for chronic low back disorders. J Spinal Disord 1996;9(4):306-12.

114. Rittweger J, Schiessl H, Felsenberg D. Oxygen uptake during whole-body vibration exercise: comparison with squatting as a slow voluntary movement. Eur J Appl Physiol 2001;86(2):169-73.

115. Clare HA, Adams R, Maher CG. A systematic review of efficacy of McKenzie therapy for spinal pain. Aust J Physiother 2004;50(4):209-16.

116. Colle F, Rannou F, Revel M, Fermanian J, Poiraudeau S. Impact of quality scales on levels of evidence inferred from a systematic review of exercise therapy and low back pain. Arch Phys Med Rehabil 2002;83(12):1745-52.

117. Dagfinrud H, Kvien TK, Hagen KB. The Cochrane review of physiotherapy interventions for ankylosing spondylitis. J Rheumatol 2005;32(10):1899-906.

118. Faas A. Exercises: which ones are worth trying, for which patients, and when? Spine 1996;21(24):2874-8; discussion 2878-9.

119. Hilde G, Bo K. Effect of exercise in the treatment of chronic low back pain: a systematic review, emphasising type and dose of exercise. Phys Ther Rev 1998;3(2):107-17.

120. Kool J, de Bie R, Oesch P, Knusel O, van den Brandt P, Bachmann S. Exercise reduces sick leave in patients with non-acute non-specific low back pain: a meta-analysis. J Rehabil Med 2004;36(2):49-62.

121. Mior S. Exercise in the treatment of chronic pain. Clin J Pain 2001;17(4 Suppl):S77-85.

122. van Tulder MW, Esmail R, Bombardier C, Koes BW. Back schools for non-specific low back pain. Cochrane Database Syst Rev 2000(2):Cd000261.

123. Rainville J, Hartigan C, Martinez E, Limke J, Jouve C, Finno M. Exercise as a treatment for chronic low back pain. Spine J 2004;4(1):106-15.

124. Smidt N, de Vet HC, Bouter LM, Dekker J, Arendzen JH, de Bie RA, et al. Effectiveness of exercise therapy: a best-evidence summary of systematic reviews. Aust J Physiother 2005;51(2):71-85.

125. van Tulder M, Malmivaara A, Esmail R, Koes B. Exercise therapy for low back pain: a systematic review within the framework of the cochrane collaboration back review group. Spine 2000;25(21):2784-96.

126. Analay Y, Ozcan E, Karan A, Diracoglu D, Aydin R. The effectiveness of intensive group exercise on patients with ankylosing spondylitis. Clin Rehabil 2003;17(6):631-6.

127. Aure OF, Nilsen JH, Vasseljen O. Manual therapy and exercise therapy in patients with chronic low back pain: a randomised, controlled trial with 1-year follow-up. Spine 2003;28(6):525-31; discussion 531-2.

128. Bentsen H, Lindgarde F, Manthorpe R. The effect of dynamic strength back exercise and/or a home training programme in 57-year-old women with chronic low back pain. Results of a prospective randomised study with a 3-year follow-up period. Spine 1997;22(13):1494-500.

129. Bronfort G, Evans RL, Anderson AV, Schellhas KP, Garvey TA, Marks RA, et al. Nonoperative treatments for sciatica: a pilot study for a randomised clinical trial. J Manipulative Physiol Ther 2000;23(8):536-44.

130. Brox JI, Sorensen R, Friis A, Nygaard O, Indahl A, Keller A, et al. Randomised clinical trial of lumbar instrumented fusion and cognitive intervention and exercises in patients with chronic low back pain and disc degeneration. Spine 2003;28(17):1913-21.

131. Cherkin DC, Deyo RA, Battie M, Street J, Barlow W. A comparison of physical therapy, chiropractic manipulation, and provision of an educational booklet for the treatment of patients with low back pain. N Engl J Med 1998;339(15):1021-9.

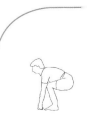

References

132. Chok B, Lee R, Latimer J, Tan SB. Endurance training of the trunk extensor muscles in people with subacute low back pain. Phys Ther 1999;79(11):1032-42.

133. Coxhead CE, Inskip H, Meade TW, North WR, Troup JD. Multicentre trial of physiotherapy in the management of sciatic symptoms. Lancet 1981;1(8229):1065-8.

134. Davies JE, Gibson T, Tester L. The value of exercises in the treatment of low back pain. Rheumatol Rehabil 1979;18(4):243-7.

135. Descarreaux M, Normand MC, Laurencelle L, Dugas C. Evaluation of a specific home exercise programme for low back pain. J Manipulative Physiol Ther 2002;25(8):497-503.

136. Fernandez-de-Las-Penas C, Alonso-Blanco C, Morales-Cabezas M, Miangolarra-Page JC. Two exercise interventions for the management of patients with ankylosing spondylitis: a randomised controlled trial. Am J Phys Med Rehabil 2005;84(6):407-19.

137. Frost H, Klaber Moffett JA, Moser JS, Fairbank JC. Randomised controlled trial for evaluation of fitness programme for patients with chronic low back pain. BMJ 1995;310(6973):151-4.

138. Ghoname EA, Craig WF, White PF, Ahmed HE, Hamza MA, Henderson BN, et al. Percutaneous electrical nerve stimulation for low back pain: a randomised crossover study. JAMA 1999;281(9):818-23.

139. Glaser JA, Baltz MA, Nietert PJ, Bensen CV. Electrical muscle stimulation as an adjunct to exercise therapy in the treatment of nonacute low back pain: a randomised trial. J Pain 2001;2(5):295-300.

140. Grunnesjo MI, Bogefeldt JP, Svardsudd KF, Blomberg SI. A randomised controlled clinical trial of stay-active care versus manual therapy in addition to stay-active care: functional variables and pain. J Manipulative Physiol Ther 2004;27(7):431-41.

141. Hagen EM, Eriksen HR, Ursin H. Does early intervention with a light mobilisation programme reduce long-term sick leave for low back pain? Spine 2000;25(15):1973-6.

142. Hagins M, Adler K, Cash M, Daugherty J, Mitrani G. Effects of practice on the ability to perform lumbar stabilisation exercises. J Orthop Sports Phys Ther 1999;29(9):546-55.

143. Hansen FR, Bendix T, Skov P, Jensen CV, Kristensen JH, Krohn L, et al. Intensive, dynamic back-muscle exercises, conventional physiotherapy, or placebo-control treatment of low-back pain. A randomised, observer-blind trial. Spine 1993;18(1):98-108.

144. Holmes B, Leggett S, Mooney V, Nichols J, Negri S, Hoeyberghs A. Comparison of female geriatric lumbar-extension strength: asymptotic versus chronic low back pain patients and their response to active rehabilitation. J Spinal Disord 1996;9(1):17-22.

145. Keller TS, Szpalski M, Gunzburg R, Spratt KF. Assessment of trunk function in single and multi-level spinal stenosis: a prospective clinical trial. Clin Biomech (Bristol, Avon) 2003;18(3):173-81.

146. Klaber Moffett JA, Carr J, Howarth E. High fear-avoiders of physical activity benefit from an exercise programme for patients with back pain. Spine 2004;29(11):1167-72; discussion 1173.

147. Langridge JC, Phillips D. Group hydrotherapy exercises for chronic back pain sufferers – introduction and monitoring. Physiotherapy 1988;74(6):269-73.

148. LeFort SM, Hannah TE. Return to work following an aquafitness and muscle strengthening programme for the low back injured. Arch Phys Med Rehabil 1994;75(11):1247-55.

149. Lewis JS, Hewitt JS, Billington L, Cole S, Byng J, Karayiannis S. A randomised clinical trial comparing two physiotherapy interventions for chronic low back pain. Spine 2005;30(7):711-21.

150. Ljunggren AE, Weber H, Kogstad O, Thom E, Kirkesola G. Effect of exercise on sick leave due to low back pain. A randomised, comparative, long-term study. Spine 1997;22(14):1610-6; discussion 1617.

151. Long A, Donelson R, Fung T. Does it matter which exercise? A randomised control trial of exercise for low back pain. Spine 2004;29(23):2593-2602.

152. Manniche C, Asmussen K, Lauritsen B, Vinterberg H, Karbo H, Abildstrup S, et al. Intensive dynamic back exercises with or without hyperextension in chronic back pain after surgery for lumbar disc protrusion. A clinical trial. Spine 1993;18(5):560-7.

153. Niemisto L, Lahtinen-Suopanki T, Rissanen P, Lindgren KA, Sarna S, Hurri H. A randomised trial of combined manipulation, stabilising exercises, and physician consultation compared to physician consultation alone for chronic low back pain. Spine 2003;28(19):2185-91.

154. O'Sullivan P, Twomey L, Allison G, Sinclair J, Miller K. Altered patterns of abdominal muscle